Unlikely Hope

What people are saying:

"Lew is a gifted and grateful storyteller. A sense of humility, peace, and quiet courage resonates throughout Unlikely Hope. Clearly, an inspiring read for all facing life's many challenges." **- Todd Martin, Former World #4 tennis player, Olympian, and Sports Executive**

"Unlikely Hope isn't just a book — it's a gut punch of perspective. Lew doesn't sugarcoat the brutal reality of cancer, despair, or the sheer unfairness of life. But here's the magic: in the middle of heartbreak, he cracks open grace, grit, humor, and this stubborn, beautiful will to live. As a woman who's built an empire by pushing through the impossible, I know resilience when I see it — and Lew's story is it, page after page. This isn't a 'feel-good' book. It's a feel-everything book. It will break you open, make you laugh, make you cry, and — if you let it — remind you why we keep showing up when life blindsides us. If you're looking for a perfect, polished, inspirational fluff piece — move along. But if you want raw humanity, fierce faith, and a masterclass in real courage, Unlikely Hope delivers. Big time." **- Gogo Bethke, Entrepreneur, Speaker, Founder of GoGet'Em Community**

"Grit, Determination, Compassion, Logophilic, multi-talented. Though Lew was 1 foot in the hole when I met him, he would always kill you with kindness. Lew is a multifaceted, highly educated, almost unbelievably experienced human. Kindest of hearts, and a mix between Charlton Heston, James Bond, and Martin Short with a touch of theologian. One of a kind. His story is nothing short of awe inspiring." **- Rick Danison, Associate Director of Performance, University of Alabama Football**

"Get ready: *Unlikely Hope* isn't a sentimental pep-talk. It's no triumphant victory lap. Rather, it's an honest, skillfully rendered account from the edge of the abyss. If you or someone you love stands there, too, I can think of no better companion than Lew Worthington." **- Sarah Arthur, cancer survivor and best-selling author of The Carrick Hall Novels**

Unlikely Hope

My Journey from Death to Life
With Pancreatic Cancer

Lewis Worthington, PhD

...they have gone from death to life.
-John 5:24

Pickled Publishing

Unless indicated otherwise, all biblical translations are the author's.

Readers may write the author or ask questions at Lew@LewWorthington.com.

Readers may follow the blog and keep up with Lew at LewWorthington.com.

Cover design by Liphus (Mick) Swindall

Published by Pickled Publishing. First Edition. Paperback.

For Abby
To Jenn

CONTENTS

FOREWORD

Few things clarify our experience of living as much as a terminal diagnosis. Understanding our mortality and the finite gift of time can lead us to moments of fear, joy, thanksgiving, and existential awe as we ponder the meaning of wisdom, faith, and love. *Unlikely Hope* is a book that compels the reader to examine the world through the lens of Lew's diagnosis, treatment, and experience with pancreatic cancer. Ultimately, it is a book about the ability to understand life in the most extraordinary circumstance.

I first knew Lew and his family as members of the church I pastored in East Lansing, Michigan. My interactions with Lew began long before his diagnosis and our relationship continued after I left the church. Learning of his illness was a heartbreaking discovery. And yet, the story of Lew's experience with cancer is not one about dying as much as it is a declaration of life. I have always known him as a vibrant, joyful, vivacious man who is full of energy and enthusiasm. Prior to his diagnosis, he had faced trials, yet he spoke of his challenges with a reflective pragmatism that demonstrated his understanding of the complexity of life in community and relationship. He faced the brutal reality of his cancer with the same realism.

Lew does not sugarcoat his fight with cancer or try to wrap up his experience with a bow made of cliché lessons of redemption. Rather, he guides the reader through his journey with humor, vulnerability, spiritual reflection, frustration, and humility. His book is relatable in that all people understand the unique moments that throw us off our course and send us on a different, unfamiliar path. While the destination may not be clear, how we travel together is an important exercise in living.

Each chapter of *Unlikely Hope* invites you to imagine how you might stand beside someone facing a similar diagnosis, treatment, or decision. It is a book that stretches our empathetic muscles and calls us to be with Lew as he asks questions, wonders about the future, and hopes in the face of uncertainty. This memoir is full of courage and compassion, even when doubt and suffering are ever present.

What makes this book exceptional isn't simply Lew's heroic battle with pancreatic cancer. It is the way he insists that hope is still possible. Hope is not just wishful thinking, but it is a practice—something grown, fought for, and carried not despite hardship, but through it. Lew has discovered great wisdom in his unlikely hope and that wisdom is here to be shared. The Hebrew and Greek words for wisdom appear in the Hebrew Bible and Christian New Testament only fifteen times less than the word love. If love is the completion of God's law, then wisdom is the practical understanding of this love in action. The wisdom Lew discovered is rooted in the love he found in his family and community in his most challenging moments.

May this story be an opportunity for you to reflect on that same love found in the unexpected wisdom discovered through Lew's miraculous story in *Unlikely Hope.*

Andrew Pomerville
President, Louisville Presbyterian Theological Seminary
May, 2025

PROLOGUE

At 6:00 PM on May 15, 2023, a text message came to me. It was from Joel Wondra, the Athletic Director at Shawano Community High School. He had read my wife's announcement on Facebook that my most recent blood test—that stressful and dreadful rite always performed as a prelude to my periodic visits with the oncologist—had indicated relative health. I could never look at the results myself. Jenn was courageous enough to soften the bad news if there were any, and joyous enough to bring glad tidings otherwise.

Three years earlier, Joel had hired me to be the school's varsity volleyball coach just as the world was in the midst of social distancing from rampant COVID-19. As a new pastor in town, I thought this would be a great way to get to know people in this community. When the team started meeting together that summer for open gym sessions, the players were forbidden to touch a ball that someone else had touched. This restriction was mandated by the state high school athletic association, and it made sense from a public health point of view, but it made volleyball seem like we had just entered some kind of sports zombie apocalypse. As with football and many other sports, the game only works when one player can successfully deliver the ball to someone else.

The season was full of other challenges. Some of the schools in our conference canceled their seasons altogether. Other matches were canceled or postponed indefinitely. Fielding a roster was also a unique problem since COVID touched so many families on our team. But the chief issue confronting our team that season had to do with another serious health matter. Two years earlier, Abby, a gifted and energetic setter who had come to Shawano to play volleyball, was diagnosed with brain cancer. After chemo, surgery, and whatever other treatments doctors prescribed along the way, her ability to compete at a high level was impaired, but not her love of the game and her spirit to play.

But Abby made our team because we needed her. We needed her expertise and her leadership. We needed her passion and I, as a coach with some college coaching experience, needed her help to figure out how to coach at this level. We attended an unofficial tournament that summer and our lineup only made sense because of my reliance upon Abby's know-how and familiarity with our team.

Abby's physical weakness made setting a volleyball difficult for her. I could tell by the way she handled the ball that hers were some of the sweetest hands I had seen among high schoolers, but her leg strength often made it impossible for her to get to the ball on time, and her feeble legs, arms, and hands made it impossible to set any but the shortest sets. But it was her courage and determination that defined our season that year, and it was to her that our season was dedicated.

When Joel's text came to me, I had just been reading about survival statistics of pancreatic cancer patients like me when treated with my particular chemo. Reading these things like the "dismal prognosis" associated with my disease had already torpedoed any attempt at buoyant optimism based on my healthy blood test. Yet, I tried to embrace my short-term health with joy and gratitude. Receiving this text, then, had the potential to brighten my spirits. However, the text ended with the announcement that Abby's battle with cancer had ended that morning. I wept for my setter, my hero, my friend.

The message carried within it the bitterest of ironies: The joy of living, the sadness of dying; the long fight ahead, the termination of the battle. Cancer forces us to understand survival not merely in terms of the experience of life, but in mathematical and statistical ways apart from the experience of life. Cancer is often like that: We attempt to live as fully as possible while "living" and "possible" oppose each other. Anyone who has dealt with cancer faces these contradictions. Abby struggled with them. Joel as Athletic Director struggled with them. This book tells the story of my struggles when cancer's contradictions spilled into my life.

1 DYING

Because I could not stop for Death—
He kindly stopped for me—
The Carriage held but just Ourselves—
And Immortality.
– Emily Dickinson, "Because I could not stop for Death"

"We'll just keep an eye on it."

Doctor Jamieson laid out his plan to care for an ache in my side that had annoyed my comfortable life for about a year. I had no reason to doubt this plan. Up to this point, any health issues were typical for guys my age to experience and then gripe about. And these complaints were always buffered with the standard "it sure beats the alternative" reminder that is supposed to keep such aches and pains in perspective.

Well, I also had a history of bad knees. I figured medical science would advance enough by the time I needed it to fix joints completely without resorting to cleavers, drills, and hammers. After three surgeries, I stayed active through a commitment not to be bored and a regular use of ibuprofen. The problem, a

physician friend reminded me, is that damage to the stomach lining could result from prolonged use. The irony is that my healthy, active lifestyle could lead to some serious health problems. "Pick your poison," he said.

Other than that, I fully expected to live for a long time. In addition to healthy lifestyle choices, I was blessed with some genes on my father's side that were unusually cooperative with the idea of longevity. My grandmother and several of Dad's siblings lived into their mid-90s in spite of a tradition of southern, home-cooked meals and all the fat and cholesterol that go along with them. Furthermore, Caleb, my youngest son, was born when I was 55, and I promised to stick around until he was at least that age. I know the years were not guaranteed, but if my dad's family members were nonagenarians without really trying, a century was worth a shot. One hundred ten is the new ninety-five.

Oddly, I always enjoyed going to Doctor Jamieson's office. Not only was it encouraging to be reminded how healthy I was, but his lobby and patient rooms were like a world sports hall of fame. The prominence of framed degrees and certifications gave way to a catalog of trophies, laminated magazine and newspaper articles, and photographs. What was most amazing is that he was featured in all of them. He had pictures with Magic Johnson, Sugar Ray Leonard, Sam Snead, Arthur Ashe, and others as if they were old friends. They probably were. He actually defeated tennis Hall of Famer Ashe in a college tennis match and bested golf Hall of Famer Snead in a golf fundraiser. He was not merely a collector of stuff; he was a curator of experience. This is a fun place to get a checkup.

The photo of Ashe reminded me of an interview the tennis great gave years after he suffered a heart attack at the age of 36. Up to that point, he confessed, he was not aware of the difference between being in shape and being in good health. I often thought about that, and how nasty it would be to dedicate your life to healthy things only to be blindsided by something like cardiovascular disease. Misfortune can do that. Genetic history can do that. But that was his story, not mine.

So, I marched toward fulfilling my promise to Caleb. I could live my life and imagine what life would be like a half century from now, even without realistically expecting to survive that long. The key was to make plans and dream of the future my entire past was preparing me for because life's next phase will always be the best one.

When I landed my dream job in Shawano, Wisconsin, it seemed the best phase had finally arrived, so it might not be completely stupid for me to forget short term discomfort to take the job. Sure, we would haul the family seven hours from the home that brought us together, the hub of our activities, my wife, Jenn's business, and our friends, but the move would take us within 35 minutes of Lambeau Field, the home of the Green Bay Packers. That is a huge factor to me—one of the biggest Packers fans never to have worn a cheesehead.

Besides, fulfilling life's God-given purpose has nothing to do with simple geography. It seemed as if the previous years of my life were to prepare me for this position, and it seemed like I had finally found my dream job, pastoring a beautiful congregation in Shawano. I was placed on this planet for this reason, and it did not matter to me where on this planet I was placed. So, we bought a house, moved most of our stuff into it, and Caleb and I began life in America's Dairyland. Jenn and her folks, who would move in with us, would join us after they tied up some loose ends in Michigan.

Before my family's arrival, our congregation, like most in the United States, struggled to maintain membership. This decline, of course, has been the subject of a bajillion studies sponsored by church organizations and other groups in America. The fact that many of these studies identify traits of social groups like "millennials", "gen x", "gen y", "gen z", and so forth indicates that these studies are trying to figure out what is wrong with everybody else. It is like the struggling restaurant who hired a polling organization to understand why people in that area do not like their awful food anymore. To me, the problem is that most congregations just do not do a good job loving people. So, my plan, upon arriving in this sleepy community, was to get to know as many people as possible and love them. It is a radical concept to some, I know, but I've always been a bit of a rebel.

So, after a couple months of Wisconsin residency and in a huge stroke of good fortune, I was hired by the local high school to coach their varsity volleyball team. I had mountains of coaching experience, and I have been enthusiastic about volleyball since my college days. But the point of securing a coaching position, besides positively affecting the lives of our student athletes, was to meet people in my newly adopted community. Meeting people where they lived had always been an effective church growth approach for me and my congregations in the past, and I was convinced we could revitalize this lovely congregation. Everything was falling into place! When things seem so right, so ordained by God to be so perfect, so blessed in so many ways, what can possibly go wrong?

*****

The call came too late to be a happy one. The color in Mom's face, neck, hands, and seemingly even her nightgown vanished. She held her fingertips up to her chin and whispered, "You're kidding." Even though I was only nine years old at the time, I knew something had gone terribly wrong somewhere. I breathlessly stared at Mom's troubled face.

The news was that my cousin, Rusty, had died. Rusty was one of three children in my dad's sister's family. Aunt Sarah and Uncle Carl and their kids had always been a warm and welcome extension to our own nuclear family. Sarah and Dad were numbers 11 and 12 in a baker's dozen of siblings who survived into adulthood from my paternal grandparents. The rest of that side of the family was not close, but we did everything together with this part of the clan: We shared all our vacations, we ate countless meals together, we holed up in a basement through a tornado, and now, unexpectedly, we shared in the grief of Rusty's death.

It was my first experience with the reality of dying. I had thought about it before. Months before Rusty's death, I wept before my older brother, John, about death. It was the first time I realized that everybody dies and that I, too, would die *some* day. I thought about my absence when everybody else I knew gathered together. That thought saddened and frightened me. John, just sixteen months older, consoled me with the thought that I would live at least into my eighties. I still wept. I vividly remember his emphatic, "But eighty years is a *long time*!" I do not think the upsetting part to my child-brain was the finite number of years we were blessed with, but that we died. Ever.

Members of my family had died before. Both sides of my family boasted robust numbers, so the census at family gatherings rivaled many villages. And with such large numbers of people, there were always old people; lots of old people who moved like old people, talked like old people, and smelled like old people. And eventually, old people die. Even in my child-brain, I realized that this was the expected result of being old. And I had lost relatives within the first nine years of my life. But they were either expected, old-people deaths, or their death happened before I was old enough to understand. But Rusty was different. He was a kid. He was one of us. His death was not expected.

I remember the funeral several days later. Even then, I did not understand how his parents or my cousins, Kathy and Greg, could live normally. What an awful thing, death. And now we were at a funeral. Ugh. When we arrived at the church, I first caught a glimpse of Rusty's body at the front of the sanctuary. Rusty looked like Rusty always looked, but now his body was no longer alive. Without realizing how uncouth it could've been, I tapped John on the shoulder, pointed forward, and lipped, "Look!" He understood social protocols better than I, so he silently turned his gaze downward and smoothly held out his hand, palm down, to subdue my discovery.

I suppose it is nearly universal to have thoughts and feelings about death. The fact that we all share this fate offers no comfort. I understand Mickey's question in the movie, "Hannah and Her Sisters" when he realizes that he will eventually die: Doesn't that ruin it for you? It could, especially if we were haunted by the "Die now, pay later" policy that Mickey mentions in the movie. But there were only a few things in life that it ruined for me. Ever since Rusty's death, which came by means of choking on a piece of steak, eating steak always has an associated fear. Likewise, I always hate getting phone calls late at night because this is how unbearable news is communicated. For many years, I could not sleep on my back because the only way to be comfortable in this position is to fold my hands on my chest. But this is how the mortician arranged Rusty's hands for display. Other than that, and other than the sadness of losing loved ones, I was much too busy living the fullest 110 years anybody ever lived.

*****

COVID isolation imposed itself one week after my family completed our move to Shawano. Along with every other human on earth, trying to grow thriving businesses in Jenn's case, or thriving faith communities in mine, had new and unexpected challenges. Through the miracle of modern medical insurance bureaucracy, it became impossible to "keep an eye" on the little ache that entered my internal organs without being invited while living in Wisconsin. But also, because of the quarantine, we found ourselves making regular round trips between our new home in Shawano and our former community in central Michigan.

During one of these trips, I scheduled an appointment with a gastroenterologist (GI), a medical doctor who specializes in human guts. She could make no determination of what caused the pain in my side and guessed that it could be something as bothersome as irritable bowel syndrome (IBS). I remember exhaling in exasperation, not embracing the idea of dealing with needling little medical problems for the rest of my long life. However, my description of the type and location of the pain did not seem to be in the right place for IBS. Plus, the lack of other symptoms made diagnosis challenging. She suggested ingesting MiraLAX on a regular basis and scheduled an appointment a few weeks out to give the treatment time to have a corrective impact.

My follow-up appointment put me in touch with a Physician's Assistant. We discussed hypotheticals since no real problem was identified. Since the location of the ache was not where IBS usually bothers a patient, what else could it be? Finally, in the pursuit of Truth, Jenn suggested a CT scan. I mean, why not? No other diagnostic procedure led to anything stronger than a guess. "OK," the PA started. "Let's do that just to make sure nothing horrible is going on."

Like other bad news in my life, it was late one Sunday night that an email came into my inbox. I had new test results in my patient portal, the message heralded. I could look at the results, and I would in spite of the disclaimer that my doctors had not seen these tests. I experienced no concern or panic as Jenn and I looked for the expected outcome of the test, which surely would be that there was nothing serious going on. What we found, however, was an indication of a growth on my pancreas that was the size of a soup can. The analysis was shrouded in medical terminology, so my immediate hope was that my ignorance was leading me to draw hasty conclusions. Still, we stared in disbelief at the computer screen. I had a momentary flashback to the time when I saw Mom grow pale at the news of Rusty's death, and I was sure my face and neck and hands had turned a whiter shade of pale.

A sleepless night followed. While hoping for a miracle that we misunderstood the test results, the only miracle we experienced was that the following day eventually came. As soon as we could, we called the clinic that was home to the previous consultations. We would like to speak with the GI. We expressed concern that my pancreas was hosting an otherworldly alien whose intent was to invade my body; that is what cancer is, after all. After several rounds with several desk employees whose duty was to shelter patients from actual life-saving information, we were angrily dismissed with, "If there's a problem, we'll get back to you! Good-bye!"

After reading the report in my patient portal, I recalled a conversation with a friend who worked with patients as a home care nurse. Many people under her care confronted cancer. I asked her what, in her experience, was the worst type of cancer among her patients. Without hesitating, she said, "Pancreatic cancer." Those words echoed in my mind then and many times over the next several months. It appeared, even without professional confirmation, that I had the worst kind of cancer.

Is this happening to me? I could be wrong, of course. I could have misunderstood the test results. Nevertheless, trusting in one's ignorance never seems like a safe bet; the report I read from the CT scan seemed pretty clear. But if there was really a problem, I had the professional assurance that the clinic would let me know. Yet, I've never depended on the rudeness of strangers.

Through the kindness of Jenn's physician, Dr. Raus, I spoke with an oncologist who was able to confirm our worst fears. I've always been curious about how professionals handle delivering bad news, especially when it becomes a routine part of their vocation. We met the cancer doctor in the cancer center in his cancer room with all kinds of cancer posters and literature around and various cancer patients gloomily awaiting their respective treatments or verdicts. The first words to come from his mouth were, "I'm Doctor Ahmad and I'm an oncologist. The reason you're seeing an oncologist is because you have cancer." His words were well practiced but his tone was compassionate.

The first order of business is to confirm through a biopsy what appeared to be conclusive evidence from the scan. My mind has always been oriented to look at things mathematically, and I wanted to know just how sure Doctor Ahmad was. Words like "very sure" or "quite positive" are far too descriptive. I wanted numbers to attach to these descriptions. "Is there any chance at all that it could be something else?" I pressed. "Can you put it in terms of percentages?"

"Maybe there's a one percent chance that it's something else."

Without intending to imitate Lloyd from "Dumb and Dumber," I expressed the reality this number represented: "So, you're telling me there's a chance?"

If there is a way to sink from dismal suspicion to completely bleak certainty, the biopsy introduced Jenn and me to this new level of despair. It did not help that the doctor who performed the analysis hid behind his lack of empathy by delivering the results before I was completely alert following the biopsy procedure, void of the human factor that Doctor Ahmad had rehearsed. If it is possible to process information while still deeply under the influence of anesthesia, I must have done it there. Jenn held me and we wept together.

The Poet Robert Frost reportedly said, "In three words, I can sum up everything I've learned about life. It goes on." But experience teaches me that always, eventually, life does not go on. And sometimes, even when it does, the adornments that add zest to living molder and fade and rust, and these changes may be too severe and too numerous to make life recognizable as the thing that we enjoyed as Life. I was apparently stepping into those changes.

2 DESPAIRING

> But don't pretend that it won't end
> In the depth of your despair
> – Elton John & Bernie Taupin, "Idol"

When I was a child, my parents bought a bright red Impala. Until we owned that vehicle, every other car on the road was just another piece of the background. But an odd thing happened when we parked that 3,000-pound candy-apple Chevrolet in our driveway: We observed that just about every car that mattered to our lives, and about half the cars that did not, were about the same color. I even remember Mom affirming that, "Half the cars on the road are red!" Or so it seemed. No other color mattered. Auto dealerships offered two choices: Red and not-red, and those two broad colors sold in equal volumes.

We've all experienced the same kind of thing: We might have a conversation about a song we have not heard in years, then over the next week, we notice the song playing everywhere. Or a celebrity whose name we learn today immediately appears in every movie that we want to see. There is a name for this kind of experience: The Baader–Meinhof phenomenon. It refers to the tendency to observe something with odd frequency once we notice it for the first time. Of course, things do not really happen with increased frequency after we learn about them, but it just seems like it.

That is what pancreatic cancer was for me. Before my diagnosis, cancer was something that happened, and I vaguely knew about some types, and that cancer is sometimes very treatable and sometimes deadly, and that early detection is important. I knew that there were lifestyle choices we could make that would reduce the likelihood of getting cancer, and that sometimes, this ridiculous disease invades regardless of our efforts. But for the most part, I knew that cancer sucked, and people either had it, or they did not have it.

There were a small number of cancer types that transcended my "cancer/no cancer" human health classification system. Maybe my eyes were more alert to lung cancer because of how often it is preventable by simply choosing not to smoke, and how many smokers there have been in my family. And maybe any kind of cancer in children held a place in my world because of how the universe makes less sense because of it, and recently because my friend, Abby, had brain cancer. And maybe some types of cancer like breast cancer and stomach cancer disrupted my simplistic classification system because members of my family were treated for these. And maybe pancreatic cancer held a special place in my observations of the world around me because of how my nurse friend categorized it as the worst kind. Plus, even before my medical verdict was announced, I was aware of the battle that Alex Trebek fought and lost to pancreatic cancer. But otherwise, people I had known or famous people whose names I knew either died of some-kind-of-cancer, or they died of not-cancer.

But after my diagnosis, the Baader–Meinhof phenomenon hit me hard. Not only Trebek, but his predecessor on TV's *Jeopardy*, Art Fleming, also died of pancreatic cancer. I learned that jazz greats, Dizzy Gillespie and Count Basie died from it. Physicist Wolfgang Pauli and mathematician Benoit Mandelbrot succumbed to it. Actors Alan Rickman and Rex Harrison, too. Ruth Bader Ginsburg, Syd Barrett, Henry Mancini, and countless other people whose names are known by many—I took note that all these people perished from pancreatic cancer after my diagnosis.

But not every victim of pancreatic cancer dies immediately after its discovery. For some people, such as Monty Python's Eric Idle, detection was early enough that the tumor was removed and he required no further treatment. I also heard about a friend of a friend who injured himself in the upper abdomen area while fishing, and in the examination after the injury, they discovered pancreatic cancer and removed the tumor. The problem for most of us is that we live without symptoms for too long and the cancer has a chance to increase its devastation.

In my case, when all the reports were in, we discovered that I had stage IV pancreatic cancer. Even without its spread into other parts of my body, surgery was not an option for me because of the tumor's encasement around the celiac artery, one of the body's main blood suppliers to the upper abdominal area. I was not one of the lucky few whose detection comes early. So, along with noticing other people who shared my diagnosis, I became acutely aware of what their prognosis was.

*****

About the same time as my diagnosis, I had read that Tim Keller, a prominent pastor in Manhattan, had also been diagnosed with stage IV pancreatic cancer. He wrote that after his diagnosis, his sensory perception became heightened: Colors seemed brighter, days seemed more beautiful, and even sex was an elevated experience.

Nothing about Keller's pastoral meditations resonated with my sensory or emotional experience. Even before treatments began, the perceptual lens through which I viewed all of reality was dark, dreary, and dull. Sleep was not restful but only happened out of necessity. Mealtimes were devoid of pleasant talk or delicious enjoyment. Sharing family time was a struggle because any laughter, any smiling, any cheerfulness, emerged only artificially as I choked back unuttered sadness.

To add to my dismal perception of reality, since the diagnosis was announced in early December, and since my insurance would only cover treatments in Michigan, and since I could no longer continue working, we were forced to abandon what was the closest thing to heaven on earth I had ever imagined: our gorgeous house in the woods of Wisconsin, leadership among some of the most loving people ever assembled as a congregation, and the privilege of coaching the best sport in the world. Making the move back during the shortest, coldest days of the year into one of the most sunshine deprived areas of the country only added to the gloom of melancholy.

Times like these are when my personal faith in God's everlasting love and the promise of eternal life probably should have kicked in. I read what Tim Keller had written and about his longing to meet Jesus and all that. Enlisting a verse from Hosea before him, the Apostle Paul asks Death where its victory and sting are, fixing his gaze to a victorious eternity in paradise. I wondered, though, if he would have taken his argument a different direction had he envisioned his body slowly being attacked by cellular invaders. My brain agreed with Paul, and with Tim Keller, and with others who embraced the promise. But the slow torment that lay ahead for me, and the prospect of leaving my Caleb behind when I had so much to share, or my Jenn whose love seemed ever fresh, or my older children, Rachel and Joshua, or my grandchildren Rosalind and Vincent, or my mom or my brothers, that is where the sting of death was for me.

I remember the first time I read the word "terminal" referring to my condition. After I resigned the position in Shawano, I read the letter to the congregation our council president had written to members of the church. I knew it—that word, "terminal"—was coming, but I had not seen it in print yet. Only Jenn and I had talked about it, what it meant, what it implied, what it felt like. All the flippant remarks I had heard or thought about that life itself is "terminal" offered no consolation.

There were many other things I faced in the ensuing months that were the first of my life. My first oncologist, my first chemo, my first baldness. Even getting my first Social Security check, which I thought would come through a celebratory retirement, came over the next few weeks. And each "first" was a bitter reminder of the new path I was on: A short, rocky, unlit path with a sign at the entrance that announced, "DEAD END".

I also developed an awareness that many things in life I had previously taken for granted might be something I was doing for the last time. I remember climbing the stairs from the basement in our house in Shawano realizing that it would be the last time I would ever do that. That kind of thing always happens when a person moves to a new residence. But I realized within weeks, perhaps, I would be climbing stairs—any stairs—for the last time. I had no idea how weak chemo would leave me, but even without a loss of strength, I just might not have much time left. I suggested to myself that the tube of toothpaste I was using might be my last. I ate a sandwich a few days before chemo was scheduled realizing that I may never eat that kind of thing again. I mulled over almost everything I did, things that have always been routine, and knew that there was a very real chance that I would not do that thing again.

*****

The days of December and January of that winter were filled with considerations of treatment options. The most reasonable choices were two types of chemotherapy. The point of doing chemo at all, originally, was to shrink the tumor enough so that surgery could be done. But when cancer was detected in the lymph nodes, surgery was no longer an option. So, then the objective became to prolong life as much as possible. Of these two choices, one had less severe side effects but only had a positive effect for about a fourth of the patients. The other choice was effective for just under half the patients, but the side effects were more severe. The words of my physician friend years earlier, "Pick your poison," rang in my ears, but with more literal accuracy than before.

Other options were out there. My wish was that some type of mRNA vaccine or immunotherapy would be developed in time to try it. We also considered clinical trials and conferred with specialists at the University of Michigan who were eager to enroll me into a Phase I trial. They were only interested in patients who had no prior chemotherapy. The point of the trial was to test an experimental drug that would be used in tandem with chemo. However, the test stipulated that the chemo used would be the milder, less probably effective form. My mathematical orientation wanted to know the statistics, the probabilities; that is, what could I reasonably expect? How many points of probable effectiveness will I sacrifice if I join the trial, as opposed to being hit with the other form of chemo without a trial drug? I wanted statistics because my life depended on these numbers. But for a Phase I clinical trial, there are no numbers. Also, Phase I trials provide solid clinical data related to dosing, namely, how much of the drug is needed to be optimal? From my point of view, it seemed as if they were interested in enrolling people who were probably going to die soon enough, and they simply wanted to make sure the doses of the experimental treatment would not kill them before the cancer did.

Ultimately, we decided on the treatment with the greater chance of effectiveness to reduce the size of the tumor. It was a pretty easy choice simply because I wanted to stack the odds in my favor as much as possible. I started asking myself how much I would give in terms of money, comfort, physical abilities, or anything else I could hypothetically put on the bargaining table, in exchange for another percentage point of possible effectiveness. It was all about the probability of the drugs working. Nothing else mattered.

*****

It is a scary thing when the nurses who handle the bags of drugs they're about to pump into your body wear a hazmat suit because touching this stuff could ruin a person. I can see why. Within minutes of my first six-hour session, my extremities started to feel tingly. The nurse in charge responded by adding some kind of medication to the cocktail that was streaming into my body. I'm not sure the new ingredient helped much. "Maybe", my subconscious self-narrated to my conscious self, "it was a placebo they administered just to see if I was inventing symptoms that didn't actually develop."

The treatments began in January. The tingling that emerged at the onset of treatments matured into an army of pinpricks instigated by any exposure to cold. Avoiding cold things in a Michigan winter—things like surfaces, water, air—is as difficult as avoiding everything, like surfaces, water, air, because everything is cold. I learned quickly that routine actions like washing my hands needed to be prepared by a ritual of running the tap until tolerable warmth was reached. I was a little disappointed in myself for not just putting up with it. *Pain is temporary*, and all that kind of heroic nonsense could not withstand this new level of torture brought on by a few degrees below room temperature.

The next sensory feature stripped of normalcy was taste. We had all grown accustomed to answering questions about a "loss of taste or smell" during the COVID quarantine. The accompanying loss of appetite paired with a shrinking ability to digest nutrients created enmity between me and one of my oldest and dearest friends: food. Of all the normal functions chemo stole from me, this was the cruelest.

When I held my first church ministry position many years earlier, the congregation's senior pastor shared details about a home visit he had with a church member whose health was failing. "He is so ill," said my mentor, shaking his head, "that he couldn't even get down the morsel of bread for communion." My pastor had a grim look on his face as we both silently questioned how a body could sink into that kind of hell. How could something so basic to life itself—or, in symbolic portions, so basic to faith—swell into an impossibility?

The next few months saw my weight drop off as I manipulated these digestive liabilities in various ways. Since I could not taste most foods, I relied on the strong taste of vinegar to involve my taste buds in the eating experience. However, spinach with vinegar does not supply enough calories to sustain life. And sauerkraut, another vinegar laced candidate, blessed me and those around me with additional atmospheric side effects.

Getting food down was an act of supreme discipline. I envied everyone around me as they enjoyed meals in spite of their love and compassion for me. I realized for the first time the central place the act of eating, not merely nourishing ourselves, occupied in our lives. In my weakened state, I watched tons of movies. It seemed as if every movie I watched featured characters talking with food in front of them. These fictional characters were not immune to my jealousy as I lusted not for the food in front of them, but for the act of eating the food implied. I even asked myself whether they got tired of eating whatever they were eating if the director ordered multiple takes.

As I continued to lose my palette, some taste sensations became repulsive. I remember one day after someone brought home some delicious looking grapes, everyone else commented on their perfect flavor. My experience, of course, was completely different. Eating these perfect fruits resembled what I imagined the dank dust in an old cellar would be like, if we could package that dust in a juicy grape-shaped seedless sack.

One protein rich food I could tolerate was sardines. It is an oddball food I've enjoyed in normal life, but chemo stripped enjoyment from the experience. Even smoked oysters in a tin, not normally regarded as fine dining, were bearable. I could not detect the oyster flavor itself and the little seafood nuggets resembled bouncy balls so eating them was like munching rubberized soot. But at least it went down and stayed down.

Vicarious eating became my favorite pastime. During many sleepless nights between rounds of crossword puzzles on my phone, I loved watching Gorton's frozen fish advertisements. There was something oddly comforting about the images and the dream of eating real frozen fish, a substance I had previously regarded as an oxymoron. I dreamed of another day, either in the past or in the future, when I could enjoy a meal. And maybe it would be an entire box of Gorton's fresh caught, frozen, battered, oven heated, whole fish filets. Heaven!

My weight continued to melt off. I sadly observed how my knees bulged out beyond the rest of my legs, and how the skin around my thighs wrinkled like an old rubber balloon after all of its air escaped naturally. When descending downstairs where the rest of my family lived became too difficult, physically and emotionally, I holed up in our bedroom and awaited whatever was next. I never dreamed of leaving this life in a blaze of glory, but after a lifetime of health and determination, this way of exiting was intolerable.

When visited by a hospice nurse, she assured me that the end may not be near, whatever "near" means. I knew she was trying to help, but it was a dose of help I did not want. In her attempts to console me in my near skeletal condition, she said, "Oh, you'd be surprised at how much weight you can lose and still be alive." That is not exactly what I needed to hear.

Eventually, the most efficient and effective substance I found for slowing down bodily erosion were these super high calorie protein drinks. As much as I hated the experience of having the best meal of the day forcing down an overly sweet concoction with the viscosity of Pepto Bismol, it seemed that this stuff was prolonging my life by a few days. Maybe a few weeks. Who knows how long? And why would I want to? It all seemed so pointless.

Jenn and I talked about ways of hastening the end of this shadow of a life. I assured her that this would certainly not be my style. I thought about Caleb in his youth, and I was curious how his life would turn out. What passions would he develop? What kind of young man will he be? I wanted to see just the next step. Then the next. Then the next. I decided I was willing to do whatever it takes just to see his life's next steps. For that, I needed a miracle.

3 QUESTIONING

As flies to wanton boys are we to th' gods;
They kill us for their sport.
– William Shakespeare, *The Tragedy of King Lear* (Act IV,
Scene 1)

We all ask questions that express emotions rather than seek answers. I once saw French American tennis pro Maxime Cressy in the midst of not playing his best game asking, *"Pourquoi?! Pourquoi?!"* ("Why?! Why?!") In many ways, I felt a deep sense of brotherhood with Cressy's struggle as it seemed nothing about his game remotely resembled normalcy. I recalled my own tennis frustrations when I questioned everything about the game I love, including why I can't hit any shot at all, why I ever started playing tennis, and why God would allow such an evil thing as tennis to be invented.

Anyone who has ever played tennis, or has ever golfed, or has ever lived in the real world has had reason to ask this question. We've all experienced real-life situations when frustration boils over into asking unanswerable questions. In those moments, the answer might be as pointless as the question.

I have often questioned cancer. Cancer is such an uncaring beast. It gives no reason, cares nothing about the outcome of its intrusion into the victim's body, and up to this point in history, conceals many of its scientific—and all its philosophical—mysteries. Still, when confronted with its insidious intrusion into our lives, we often pointlessly and emotionally ask, "Why?! Why?!"

A few days after my initial diagnosis, Jenn and I found ourselves in deep embrace sharing the pain and weeping out that small, grievous word: Why? The science in my background was sufficient for me to recognize the futility of the interrogation. In the awareness that I did not fit the profile of typical pancreatic cancer victims, I asked Why; it just looked like "bad luck" as one of my oncologists put it. Then the theology in my background protested even stronger with the same refrain: Why?

There is a massive history of people asking about suffering in the world. Many religious traditions have expressed solutions to the problem. Perhaps some god or devilish imp is out there hell-bent (literally) to damage us. Maybe in God's loving, infinite wisdom, having people suffer randomly (it seems) results in love and compassion in ways that would otherwise not happen. I've studied this topic deeply and even wrote a paper about it, but all that learning and all those theories do not matter much when you're suffering without an answer to the *why* question.

Sometimes, this riddle is expressed this way: Why do bad things happen to good people? Back in olden times when people were apparently much less loving and stupider than they are today, there was a lot of finger pointing and tongue wagging, and the assumption was that the victim or someone in the victim's family did something terribly wrong, like they forgot to pay their tithe or they noticed the comeliness of some fair maiden or their brother's family lusted after the neighbor's swimming pool. But I never claimed to be a good person, so the conundrum of bad things happening to good people did not apply to my deadly cancer.

There were always people who seemingly deserved that kind of fate even less. Abby was a gifted athlete who was doing a great job of enjoying her early high school years when brain cancer derailed all attempts at a normal life. I met Abby when I was installed as volleyball coach at the high school in my newly adopted community. It did not make sense to anyone. Why can't she live the lovely, happy, long life that God surely intended for her to live? Even before my own diagnosis, I uttered the *Why* question to God, not so much expecting an answer as to express my frustration about a world governed by a loving God that simply did not make any sense.

Just because these questions cannot be answered, and just because the answers, even if we had them, would not help, that does not stop people from offering their two cents. And really, at two cents it is usually not worth the money. It does not happen often, because most of the people who are courageous enough to talk to somebody who is dying of cancer have enough love and concern that they understand the limited market value of empty platitudes. Yet, there are still those willing to shovel out popular wisdom at bargain basement prices. If "nobody said life is fair" doesn't heal a troubled heart, you might get "it is what it is" in a buy-one-get-one-free sale. (By means of rebuttal, I distinctly remember hearing someone say that life *is* fair—even if it isn't—and I can also counter with the fact that "it isn't what it isn't". Whew. I feel better.)

I get it. As Abby shared near the end of her life, many of her former friends started to drift away simply because they could not bear the awkwardness of owning a quiver of verbal cures that was completely empty. And sometimes, just because something is true does not mean the words should be spoken. People who proudly proclaim their bluntness are masking behind their acute lack of tact and sensitivity. Sometimes, we just want concern and some kind of assurance that at some point in somebody's past, we mattered. We do not need words.

We do not need too much visitation, either. At least for me, I was more quickly running out of social capital than ever when I was in the deep sludge of the chemo experience. Plus, I did not have the heart to just ask people to leave. Although at one point, when I was always sleepy, one conversational partner regaled me with stories of his glorious, happy childhood even while I was growing increasingly aware of my own snoring. With the tiny bit of consciousness I had remaining, I attempted to snore more loudly as a way of delivering a hint. But he kept the tales firing at me, stopping only long enough to reload. "Screw it," I thought to myself as I drifted off.

*****

German philosopher Friedrich Nietzsche suggested that pain and pleasure are so tied together that to experience the greatest possible joy, we must also experience the greatest possible pain. If Nietzsche lived life successfully, I might have looked to him for answers to the *why* question. I suppose it is easy to see why he went off the rails in his last decade or so; life would be hard if you thought the best you could do in the joy department is break even. My dad always teased that some people liked to beat their head against the wall because it feels so good when the pain stops. But is that the only way to achieve joy?

Nietzsche's idea may not provide an answer to the *why* question as much as it lowers one's expectation for a great life based on how reality is configured. Popular wisdom seems to glom on to the notion that there is some pain/pleasure bank account instituted by God or nature or humanity, and that there may be significant penalties for early withdrawal. Lots of people say, maybe without truly believing it, that "everything happens for a reason." Maybe that is partially true in that almost everything happens *because of* a reason, but it is a tough belief indeed to believe every bad thing happens *so that* misfortune's victims will reap some kind of benefit.

I always thought that a helpful attitude toward misfortune is to embrace it and grow from it. The athlete's maxim, "No pain, no gain," has grown to meme status within the general population and can be applied to any situation in life. It is potentially a great approach, counting on that moment later in life when I can benefit from my current suffering. But that only makes sense when there is a "later".

When I was continually bedridden, watching too many old black and white gangster movies, I thought of the cliche where bad guys issue a warning to their enemies that they will "teach them a lesson" by knocking them off. "It's only a lesson," I chuckled ironically, "if they can apply their knowledge later." Again, once you're dead, there is no benefit for the high cost of that style of education.

That is where I was after my initial diagnosis and during the trying days of chemotherapy: All pain, no gain. No joy to feel after the suffering. No joyful withdrawal from the pain/pleasure account despite massive misery deposits. If all I expected from God was an explanation of how this fit into a master plan for my life, God's return would've been a blank stare.

I finally decided to stop asking the *why* question.

*****

I grappled with other questions. What now? How much time do I have? What happens when it is all over? Most immediately, though, I questioned what can or will God do for me in these final moments?

For answers, I looked for gold in the deep mines of thousands of years of thinking about the human condition. My own Christian tradition affirms God's activity in the world while simultaneously exhibiting a deep, odd suspicion in any claims that we can truly see that activity. And to be honest, I've probably been the same way. Years ago, a friend was telling the story of someone she knew who had walked with a limp from childhood and how everyone in some church meeting decided to pray for healing. My friend said that she witnessed the size and shape of her irregular leg change before their very eyes and how she walked "normally" from that point on. I was not there, so how could I refute her testimony? But inwardly, I'm thinking all manner of sarcastic rebuttals, attributing what happened to the healed person to various psychological adjustments or misunderstandings. After all, coordinating the migration of a billion live bodily cells in separate paths seemed a bit too much to ask, even for our God, maker of heaven and earth.

So, I almost always regarded specific accounts of actual, physical miracles with a healthy helping of distrust. But ironically, maybe for intellectual reasons, I believed in the possibility of miracles, and even prayed for such things when loved ones needed an adjustment to reality. In principle, I believed in miracles—real miracles, not just explaining away what we do not understand. The whole idea that "the sun rising in the morning," and "the beauty of a newborn baby," and "the healing of a broken relationship" are all miracles somehow misses the point. If those are miracles simply because they're awesome, then so is the fact that my family's vacation stays within budget. Well, maybe *that* is a miracle, now that I think about it.

Naturally, the question sprouted up: Can I hope for a miracle? Beyond issues of personal belief or intellectual credibility in miracles, I had serious practical problems with it. I knew from the start of my battle that if miracles were doled out based on merit, I would be near the end of the line. I'm not pretending a false humility regarding my own candidacy for sainthood, but let's face it, children with life threatening illnesses deserve it more. For me to snatch up a nature bending exception to normalcy while a high school sophomore fights for her life seems like I jumped the line.

I'm not even talking about *expecting* a miracle. Too many lives have been damaged where a healthy and reasonable course of healing or corrective medical action was denied because the victim of illness (or worse, a minor's parents) expected God to obey their demands for a miracle. Instead of expecting a miracle, I was merely asking if a miracle is something that I could even put into my world of consideration. If it did not happen, even thinking about it might even be able to enrich me spiritually.

Almost without exception, my pastor friends encouraged me strongly to abandon such thinking. Even my new best friend in Shawano insisted on the impossibility of escaping my horrible plight through landing on a miracle. "I can't pray for a miracle," she said, "but I will pray for God's amazing comfort as Life leaks away."

I understand the reluctance to give false hope. As positive as I am by nature, I know the importance of managing expectations. Maybe it is as a safety measure that we want to see God as someone who under promises and overdelivers. If we truly believed God *always* healed our physical problems, that insurance was *always* a good value, that our judicial system *always* ruled fairly and impartially, our disappointment would be deep and disturbing when it did not happen. As it is, clinging to the promise of an immeasurable feature of God's grace such as "comfort" and "presence"—even if we know they're real—is a much more manageable expectation.

But I was not ready to dismiss the idea of a miracle, at least in principle. Two insights reinforced my confidence in keeping the concept around. First, I was listening to a lecture by a New Testament scholar whose work I admired, Craig Keener. He comes from a more conservative approach than mine and his conclusions are often vastly different from mine, but the depth of his research is peerless. Regardless of my disagreements with his interpretations, I have found his scholarship to be solid and refreshing. His "left-brained" orientation of doing work is something that resonates well with my own way of doing scholarship. At one point in his lecture, he addressed the idea of miracles in the modern world. There was no ranting on the faithlessness of miracle non-believers, no emotional departure of clear thinking. Rather, he matter-of-factly described an occasion when he witnessed the unexpected disappearance of a tumor from the body of someone he knew. I surprised myself as I found myself relating to his story on many levels. Perhaps God *is* willing to reroute billions of bodily cells after all.

The second insight may seem silly, and it probably is. But remember that I'm merely trying to build a way of looking at my vanishing life in its new context. I was reading the biblical story of King Hezekiah and how he unexpectedly fell ill and was told that he needed to get his affairs in order because he would die and that he would not recover, an announcement expressed using a typical biblical redundancy that resonated with my dismal prospects. These details were exactly mine! But there is more: Hezekiah wept and prayed and essentially told God that an early death did not make sense given his earlier life choices. That is what I did, too! For this King, God immediately heard his prayers and communicated that he would be given fifteen more years of life. I looked at my situation and imagined that an additional fifteen years would be great. It would not take me to the age of one hundred ten, but it would still be awesome!

I decided this would be my "paradigmatic narrative." This phrase is as silly as conscripting Hezekiah's story as my own, but here is what I mean: Some home builders display new homes by showing "model homes." If you have seen the series, "Arrested Development," you know what I mean. You can see what the homes look like, but you cannot actually buy them. That is what Hezekiah's story was for me: A model of recovery from a terminal illness that might give me something I desperately wanted: A future.

*****

A few weeks after chemo infusions ended, I was scheduled for a treatment called targeted radionuclide therapy. The process involved inserting my body into a long tube, and while there, expelling as much air from my lungs as possible while these amazing and sophisticated machines fired radiation right at my tumor. The hope is that the radiation will damage the DNA of the cancer cells while avoiding damage to the healthy cells as much as possible. They required me to lie as still as possible while their machines leveraged a three-dimensional picture of my insides to hit the target as accurately and effectively as possible.

I will share other details of this experience later, but two areas of reflection emerged during these treatments. First, before they could start these treatments, they needed to mark my body with two or three tattoo dots. To me, they look like I accidentally fumbled a fine tipped Sharpie on my chest. And side. And that may be all. But it was enough of an issue that someone, somewhere thought it was a clever idea to require a legally binding waiver saying that this little dot pair, the size of a small mole, would be an acceptable drawback in exchange for an attempt to save my life. Despite my physical condition, I remember laughing aloud at the absurdity of such a concern while I blurted out, "Who the heck cares?" Even for someone who is overly particular about superficial features of their image, to worry about a couple Sharpie dots seemed especially bizarre. I would just like to live, and that was a small price to pay.

Second, while the machine slowly conveyed me into the tube, these wonderful technicians outfitted me with nonmetallic earbuds through which I could listen to the music of my choice. I always found the symphonies of Gustav Mahler to promote meditation, and even though the sound equipment they provided was not high-resolution audio, it was enough for me to ponder the huge, sweeping questions of my own life. What, now, is most important? How do I want my final months to play out? What can I do to affect the world in ways that will last? I resolved then, and in the next few months, that I need to be more fully committed to other people, to be more patient toward them, to honor them with greater understanding and compassion, and to be more generous with my time and resources.

4 CARING

"Curtsey while you're thinking what to say, it saves time."
– Lewis Carroll, *Through the Looking-Glass, and What Alice Found There*

The move back to Michigan confined our entire family to a tiny house Caleb referred to as "The Shoebox". There was really nothing wrong with The Shoebox, but we associated our life together there as the end of all things. I'll admit that we as a family, or that I as an individual, did not do a good job of redeeming most of our remaining days together. We tried, but it was hard.

One of the activities Caleb and I had always enjoyed together was a periodic round of "Dive Catches". In the Shoebox, however, we elevated this periodic activity to a nightly ritual. To play this game, I would toss a small ball or pillow just above the bed, and Caleb would dash into the bedroom, dive over the mattress, and make the highlight reel worthy catch. As he matured into the longish, athletic eight-year-old he became while living in The Shoebox, he added flips, dive-rolls, and various other acrobatic ornaments to the Dive Catch experience. My job as primary ball/pillow tosser was to toss the balls almost—but not quite—out of reach. My job as Dad, though, was to keep pretending that this was the most enjoyable thing I had ever done even under the pall of cancer's death sentence.

A box arrived shortly after my diagnosis. The package, large enough to hold a bushel of apples, bore a warning not to open until further notice. Fear of punishment for noncompliance was mitigated by hearts and smiley faces adorning the message. I learned two days later that the package was the subject matter of a video conference call engineered by Abby in Wisconsin. The package rescued me from continuous sadness.

Abby's package and accompanying call provided unexpected joy and relief. She gathered up most of Shawano's volleyball team who had played under me, including members of the varsity and two junior varsity teams, to show their support. They knew what Abby had gone through, and they showed up to support me in my time of need. During our conversation, we talked about life and volleyball, but the central theme of the talk was Abby offering herself as my "chemo mentor" and describing how to use each of the gifts in the box to make treatments as comfortable as possible. There were books, movies, a blanket, a "Love Your Melon" hat, and a signed volleyball. Also, all these young student athletes wore T-shirts with letters that testified to their support proclaiming, "We're all in!" They included one of these shirts for me in the box as well. To this day, it is my favorite T-shirt, and I remember Abby and the team whenever I wear it.

What Abby masterminded that day ranks as the kindest gift I have ever received from a friend. But it did not stop there. A couple weeks later, she shared the link of a live stream of a meet the school's swim team would host. "You'll want to watch this," she promised. I was not sure why. I knew some of the kids on the swim team, but it is always hard to make out athletes' identities on video and even what event is taking place without some level of commentary.

On the night of the competition, I faithfully followed the link to the meet and quickly realized Abby's meaning. Through Joel Wondra, the school's athletic director, and the coaches and athletes on the swim team, they dedicated the competition to support me. Sharing a phrase with my favorite T-shirt, there were various posters throughout the natatorium proclaiming, "We're all in!" That makes sense, I thought, since it is impossible to swim unless you are *in* the water. But other posters specified their meaning with words of support like "We're behind you, Coach Worthington!" and "Be Strong, Coach Worthington!"

*****

Many years earlier, on a blustery day in my hometown, I was out for a bicycle ride. When I ride, I do not know how to ride casually. Even if I use a bicycle as transportation, I arrive at my destination as a sweaty mess. On this particular ride, the bluster was fully in my face. Every attempt to make this ride enjoyable and casual was circumvented by a momentum killing blast of air into my face. The six-mile stretch at the end of that day's 20-mile trek promised no relief. Besides, I was out of water, and temperatures were way too hot for enjoyment.

I recall growing grumpier and grumpier along the way, cursing the wind whose only response was pizza oven-like blasts of air into my face. Why did I take this ride? Why does the wind hate me? This is all so stupid. Stupid bike. Stupid ride. Stupid, stupid wind!

At one moment, I saw another bicyclist heading toward me. Lucky guy with the wind at his back. His path is probably all downhill, too! But I pedaled on knowing that stopping was pointless; I had to get home. I kept glancing at the distant image of the rider who was surely ridiculing me for my drudgery. I grunted on just as he, no doubt, effortlessly sailed toward me. His image grew closer and closer. I studied him as his appearance became more detailed. Then as we came within a few feet, I looked up into his face. He smiled and said, "Hi!"

That smile, that gesture of kindness somehow flipped the toggle switch of my mood. It is impossible for me not to return the pleasantness. It is also impossible for me to smile and greet someone without authentic cheer behind it. As my smile grew, so did my indebtedness to this anonymous rider. I lost the envy I had toward the rider who had powerful winds to aid rather than hinder his efforts. It was no longer a matter of weather and forces and physics and effort. It was an act of human kindness that propelled me with joy through the end of my journey.

I learned an important lesson that day. If such an easy thing as smiling can dramatically improve someone else's day, we should do more of those small acts of kindness. I realize that not all souls will be so radically blessed by something as inexpensive as a smile, but in the global economy of happiness, it seems like a worthwhile investment.

*****

When the congregation heard the news about my cancer diagnosis, many people reached out with words of love and assurance of continued prayer. Many denominations require pastors and members of the congregation to officially stop communicating with each other once new leadership takes over at the church. My denomination, as obsessed as we are with process and protocol, is no exception to this rule. I realized in the final weeks of my position at this church that we were entering into our final conversations and our final expressions of mutual support. But I knew many of them would pray. I knew some would talk and inquire about my condition and I knew I would pray for them and wonder about their future.

Support poured in from countless others whose love, concern, and faith were more than I deserved. Relatives and friends, friends of relatives, and relatives of friends all professed support through prayers or good thoughts or good vibes or any mixture of those soothing ingredients. People who had only known me for a short time reached out with encouragement and deep concern. Ron, who organizes a local charitable tennis tournament for the American Cancer Society supported me with, "Lew, I'm praying for you *every day. Every single day.*"

There were other acts of kindness. Friends and family brought food, my old roommate in college sent a kit of tea, my former pastor who had recently taken up baking brought lovely loaves of bread, and many old friends whom I often thought about reconnected. Social media can be a burden at times, but there might be no better tool at keeping us connected when webs of friendships become unmanageable.

As the winter days melted into spring, I took Caleb to the park to watch him play. He was always so comfortable meeting other kids of the same age, plus or minus one hundred percent, and on this occasion, he met two boys whose COVID-19 masks could not hide their joy in playing together. While watching the boys enjoying new friendships, I started talking with their mother. She was earnest as a parent and thoughtful as a conversationalist. As we chatted, we explored raising kids, family, and life. After the subject matter migrated to the cancer that would surely end my life, she asserted something that, at the time, was such a non sequitur, She said, "That cancer is done. There's no use for it any longer. It doesn't belong." It did not make logical sense to me, and it did not resonate with anyone's experience that I knew about. But the simplicity of the statement, coming from someone so confident, would become a mantra to me in the days ahead.

Trying to be optimistic, Jenn and I sought opportunities for great experiences. We had planned to travel to Greece, but overseas experiences were vetoed by my oncologist; the order was to make no long-term travel plans because I would not live long enough to make the trip. So, we flew to Boston on a whim. Ben Zander (Jenn's favorite orchestral director) was conducting a symphony by

Mahler (my favorite composer) and we would probably never have another chance to hear such an ideal combination. I remember noticing the bustle of the crowds at the airport, silently suppressing my envy of those who see their travel as just another trip rather than a bucket list fulfillment. Then, while waiting in a security line, we met an energetic man about my age who captured us with his friendly smile. He told us that he was grabbing as much life as possible because he did not know how much time he had left. "You see," he continued, "I was diagnosed with pancreatic cancer. I was lucky enough to have surgery, but I now want to enjoy every moment. And I'm off to see the world!" We shared my situation, too, and we embraced and promised mutual prayers as he strode off to his next destination. Jenn and I stared at one another, grinning, silently wondering the same thing: Is this an angel? Because this was the injection of joy that we both needed for the journey ahead.

*****

Meanwhile, Shelly, my administrative assistant at the church in Shawano, kept in touch with me. While denominational policy ominously forbade continued relationships with congregational members, she and I were both technically staff. She sent cards on a monthly basis and occasionally called. She assured me that she would pray every single day until the cancer vanished. If strength of belief and faithfulness to a task assured results, I had nothing to worry about.

However, contrary to a commonly held belief, it does not work that way. People aren't stupid—again, contrary to a commonly held belief—and if successful prayer requests correlated perfectly to effort, then prayer would happen much more frequently. But giving specific inputs and confidently expecting certain outcomes is the realm of silicon and technology. Somehow, praying faithfully and earnestly without guaranteed success is more virtuous and more loving and more spiritual. But I have no idea how that works.

Sometimes, the difficult thing is not when your pleading goes seemingly unheeded; indeed, it is most problematic when God actually seems to intervene at your time of need, but someone else's requests are denied. I lived for a short period in northeastern Ohio. Many in this rural community struggled to make ends meet as the blight of unemployment consumed the workforce. One young man stood up in a church meeting and thanked God for the blessings in his life since, as he explained, "Many folks don't have any job, but I have two! Praise God!"

I could not rejoice with him because my heart ached too much for the "many folks". It is not just the uncertainty of the answer that makes prayer difficult, but when your prayers are answered perfectly, what then? I know too many people who are hurting or who do not recover to rejoice completely. I will continue to pray, but I will pray while looking at the plight of others.

I was puzzled by my own inconsistency. I wanted to be in a position, some day in the future, to celebrate a miraculous victory. At the same time, I knew of no other wars against inoperable pancreatic cancer where the disease surrendered. I'm sure it has happened, but I do not know those stories. Besides, my goal was not really an overall victory, but I simply hoped to evade death one day at a time. I knew that I would not win these daily contests forever, but I hated the idea of letting cancer win. And yet, as thankful as I was that people were praying for me, I knew of so many people whose prayers for prolonged life were unheeded. Even some folks who were offering petitions on my behalf suffered the loss of a loved one in similar situations.

Plus, I'm always embarrassed to ask people to do anything for me. Even with my life in the balance, I do not want to trouble other people with my concerns. Paul asked the Roman Christians in the first century to struggle with him in their prayers on his behalf. At first blush, this seems like a request that could have benefitted from the preparatory "I don't want to impose, but...." Asking people to pray for me is difficult for a variety of reasons. It is not like I'm asking them to send money or help clean my house's crawlspace. But praying is something that some people will actually do. And when that level of attentive love for me enters into their lives, it is very humbling.

*****

Chemo hit hard. I started to believe that the poisons they were pumping into my body were strategically designed to make me embrace the hope that its remedial powers failed because of the misery they ushered into my daily life. "Quality of life" became a standard topic of conversation, and my assessment always covered the range from bad to worst. In addition to loss of appetite and a dominating nausea that blocked my attempts to eat, there were other problems. Without adequate food intake, as my weight plummeted, my waning strength limited my ability to carry on normal life activities. Additionally, my nervous system was taking quite a whipping. Almost immediately, my sensitivity to cool temperatures brought on profound discomfort. Those way-too-long moments of waiting for warm water to come out of our faucets became a required time investment if I expected to drink or wash my hands. I was warned about this possibility, as well as the neuropathy that eventually affected my fingers, feet, toes, and shoulders. As an athletic kind of fellow used to making fine motor skill adjustments based on where my body parts are in a particular moment, I experienced a new level of clumsiness because of my inability to tell exactly where my body parts were at any specific moment.

As a result of the side effects, my oncologist ordered a reduction in the dosage for each infusion. I was sad to hear this since I knew a reduction of dosage implied a corresponding loss in the treatment's effectiveness. I remember his words, "You're experiencing neuropathy, and we can't have that." I inwardly screamed, "Why not? It makes no sense to keep my body intact and functioning for the sake of taking an impeccable corpse with me into death!" I was willing to lose all my limbs if I could kill this evil malignant mass!

Somehow, over several months of treatments, there were signs that the chemo was doing its job. CT scan results showed that my soup-can-sized mass was shrinking, and the blood test indicator that suggested pancreatic cancer almost six months earlier had gone down from jaw-droppingly high to about ten percent of jaw-droppingly high. Additional good news came in the form of an announcement that radiation therapy could take place and might do some more damage to that accursed tumor.

I mentioned earlier that my time in the radiation tube, a challenge even for the most disciplined claustrophobe, afforded me the opportunity to focus on life's big questions. But my ability to find enough peace in my heart to focus on anything meaningful was due largely to the kindness of the technicians, Beau and Shannon, and the radiation oncologist, Doctor DiCarlo. Several days before receiving treatment, I was placed into the tube while they shot X Rays through my belly to determine the location and orientation of the tumor. Digestion had been a monumental challenge in the days before, and they could not get a good look at it because of all the surrounding gas. I do not know why, but the idea that I was overly gaseous inspired awful feelings of being inadequate. Maybe I interpreted the doctor's opinion as an omen that therefore, they would not be able to target the tumor accurately and that it would end my life sooner than if I had kept the gas under control. Or maybe it was that my excellence at methane production implied that I'm a very amateurish digester of food. Whatever the reason, my face showed that I felt defeated. But then Dr. DiCarlo looked at me with noble understanding and kindness, patted me on the shoulder and said, "That's OK. We'll get what we need." I doubt he will ever know how much that meant to me.

Those words, and the sympathetic tone of his voice assured me that I did not unwittingly end my life months too soon through improper digestive techniques. The technicians joined in the chorus of support. Even though my body attempted to protest the whole procedure in other ways—my weakened state made it difficult to get into a supine position (that is, lying on my back); but Beau and Shannon emphasized that they would cast no judgment regarding my physical ineptitude. I will never forget their kind emotional support.

Their care put my mind and body in the mood to cooperate. After a few weeks, we could see that the radiation hit the desired target and was supplying further effectiveness against my body's carcinogenic marauders. Slowly, the mass went from the size of a 10.5-ounce blob of concentrated cream of mushroom soup to something small enough to be reported in millimeters. As my cancer shrunk and my time away from chemo lengthened, my general health started to improve.

I do not know how or why all of this was happening. As puzzled as I had been about why cancer chose me as a recipient of its sinister invasion, I was equally perplexed how both treatments had been so effective against all odds. As I said earlier, I had given up asking "why" questions, but I did not need to know why. And other than my natural, scientific curiosity, I did not need to know how any of this was taking place, either.

Still, several things became certain to me. First, even in the absence of answers to "why" or "how" questions, I am more confident than ever that the dichotomy that pits belief in God against a reliance upon science is ridiculous and pointless. Did God miraculously heal me and restore my health? I don't know. But I am convinced that my faith in God did not lead me to ignore forms of medical treatment as a sign of that faith.

Second, despite the heavy dose of technology taking aim at my insides, none of that lovely intelligence would have made any positive difference without the active care of many people. Jenn, Shelly, Beau, Shannon, Abby, Dr. DiCarlo, Dr. Raus, and countless others created a situation in which treatments could take root and become a potent weapon against my cellular enemy. Indeed, despite a pretty clearcut result from my first CT scan, the rudeness of the front desk of the clinic that ordered the scan very nearly led to a much more rapid and much more dire outcome.

Special moments have dotted the canvas of the last few years of my life resulting in a pointillistic painting that Seurat would be proud of. Parts of this painting are joyous; others are sad. I remember the first time I read the word "terminal" in reference to my condition, but I also remember seeing the phrase, "in remission" adorning my report of a routine colonoscopy. This happened soon after all other medical signs suggested I would not be around for a colonoscopy ever again. So, we used magnets to display that report, on our fridge, along with a lovely photo of my colon. And none of these dots of good news would have happened if not for science, if not for the grace of God, and if not for the goodness of loving people.

The point of sharing, listening, praying, and caring is not to engage in austere acts of self-denial. Nor is the opposite true, namely, that it can make us feel good inside, although that is a nice bonus. The point is that without kindness and sharing with one another, nothing else in life really works, and none of the rest of it really matters. It does not make any sense to me how many people live their lives with rude behavior as a standard operating procedure. Do not waste my time or anyone else's time with rudeness. Instead, be kind. It saves time.

5 HOPING

"... hope does not disappoint us..."
– Romans 5:5

On a sticky August afternoon, in the middle of our annual visit to Mom's side of the family in the thumb of Michigan, my Uncle Kent and my sports-resistant brother, John, played a softball game against my younger brother, Jeff, and me. Although Kent was only about a year older than John, the senior member of my parents' three sons, he was by far the strongest and most skilled. Jeff and I aspired to be competent players, but at nine and fourteen, respectively, we were outmatched in strength and skill.

I can understand why two-on-two softball is not covered on any of the sports networks. But Kent engineered special rules to make it a game: Force outs could be secured by the defense if they successfully gave the ball to the pitcher before the runner reached first base. Also, we split the field into regions so that balls could only be safely hit to left field, and any ball past the third pine tree was an automatic out. Still, despite these restrictions, as Jeff and I came to bat in the bottom of the third, we were being whipped by the demoralizing score of 18 to 4.

This would be our final inning since dinner was announced from Grandma's farmhouse across the dusty gravel road. Oh, great. How can we launch a comeback with only three more outs? In the absence of effort, whining seemed like a worthy strategy, which both Jeff and I exercised fully. I do not want to say that we gave up, but we certainly did not think trying was worth our trouble since we thought that we had no hope of winning. To make matters worse, we began the bottom of the last inning with two quick outs.

But the inning was not over. To our surprise, we started an impressive two-out rally. One of the special rules to compensate for a short batting lineup is to put a "ghost" runner on base when it is our turn to bat. I vividly remember loading the bases over and over while our bats found spots for the ball to move us—and our ghost runners—around the diamond. Our run total continued to swell as Kent's and John's assured victory started to fade.

What rings most soundly in my memory about that August day was not that we fell short by two runs. Rather, it was the sting of falling short after such a miraculous comeback, and that loss may have been avoided had we put forth more effort in the early part of the last inning. Whatever psychological and emotional foibles I might reveal by saying this, I confess that I felt this sting for many months afterwards. If there is a silver lining to this experience, though, it is that I learned an important lesson that followed me for the rest of my life: Giving up, even in the face of hopelessness, is supremely pointless.

The German expression that reminds us that "Hope dies last" ignores the masses of people who quit trying too early. For most, hope dies long before chances of success flicker out. Otherwise, we would not be inspired by heroic efforts in the face of *almost*—but not completely—impossible odds. I'm reminded of what tennis great Rafael Nadal said when asked why he keeps trying in matches that he will surely lose. "But if you give up, you're going to lose 100% [of those matches]." Sure, Nadal can win 10% of those, but even mere mortals always have a chance as long as we keep trying with everything we've got.

Hope is the seed of determination. Even though determination does not guarantee a favorable outcome, a lack of determination usually assures failure. This is especially true when life itself is in jeopardy. The vital importance of hope—and the devastation of hope's disappearance—has been famously documented by Austrian psychiatrist and holocaust survivor, Viktor Frankl. In his book, *Man's Search for Meaning*, he describes how prisoners did not survive the concentration camps without hope. Prisoners with the hope of eventually being freed survived more often than those who had lost hope. Furthermore, their determination was bolstered by the belief that their spouse or children would see them again if they could survive their current hell. Without hope, death was certain.

So, should we create a future fantasy to replace an almost certain reality? It sort of worked for me. I described earlier my adoption of Hezekiah's extra fifteen years of life as my model narrative. Every society across the centuries has inspired and defined its character and flavored its future based on stories its people could identify with. For me, it was not that Hezekiah was someone I could identify with, nor did I believe that God was so pleased with me that I was granted another fifteen years of life. Instead, this story was a framework I could plug possibilities into. If I only had a chance, even if it is a small one, it just might be enough to keep me going.

The difference between having little hope and having no hope is a distinction that floats in a sea of numbers. My lifelong love of math and logic, things that give most people a ticket to slumberland, means that my spirits are lifted when I see that there is a mathematical chance of success. I'm reminded of the question

Sherlock Holmes asked his friend, Dr. Watson. "How often have I said to you that when you have eliminated the impossible whatever remains, *however improbable*, must be the truth?"

I mentioned earlier that my choosing between one form of treatment or another boiled down to statistics. I wanted to know what my chances were based on previously studied results. Medical researchers know these numbers well. But often, medical science does not understand *why* treatment "A" works on some patients, but "B" does not, but "B" works on other patients and "A" does not. It would be helpful if I could build a solid case for choosing one treatment over another because of who I am as an individual, but research is sometimes primitive in that regard. So, my choices are often based on the statistics known from the general population. My dear friend Abby was so fed up with chemo in her battle, and its inability to stop the spread of cancer in her body, that she sought other *medical* treatments. Her treatments were based on methods that have demonstrated effectiveness in other situations. Unfortunately, these treatments did not help her.

Some people try weird things in the face of hopeless medical conditions, which is very Sherlock Holmes like. I heard about a man whose condition was not helped by known medical science, so he began a regimen of bathing with and drinking his own urine. There are no studies that I'm aware of that suggest any real chances of this treatment working for anything except determining the level of commitment of one's friends and family. But when every other treatment has failed, some patients consider solutions that have no known history of success.

But when I think about those numbers, I start to realize how *hope* is such a mathematical concept, at least for me. My hope is most optimistic when there are treatments that almost always work. The stubbornly awful reality with inoperable pancreatic cancer is that there are currently no treatments that will *probably* work. Whatever those slim chances are, I'll cling to choices that enhance my survival, whatever that means. In this context, it is very specifically defined by statistics and probability—even if favorable chances are very small.

Slim possibilities tarnish shiny optimism, but I found myself clinging to whatever chances I had, provided they were real mathematical chances. That thin line between impossible and miraculous was sometimes enough to keep me going. But most people do not think about the difference or need to. When Lewis Carroll's Alice found herself confronted with the Queen who invited her to close her eyes and believe the impossible, she laughed. "There's no use trying," she said: "one can't believe impossible things." The Queen's reply seems like an oxymoron: "I daresay you haven't had much practice. When I was your age, I always did it for half an hour a day. Why, sometimes I've believed as many as six impossible things before breakfast." The genius of Carroll's dialog explores both the relationship between belief and logic as well as that thin line between impossible and unlikely.

Like Alice, I was incapable of believing in impossible things even with much practice. But I took comfort in realizing that most of my life, probability never seemed to favor me, and so luck—or probability—really owed me one. I remember discussing my cancer with a specialist at the Rogel Cancer Center in Ann Arbor. As I mentioned earlier, I expressed frustration that I did not fit the lifestyle or health profile of the "typical" pancreatic patient. I was not looking for answers as much as understanding. His reply that it was just bad luck offered no comfort.

So, my older son, Josh, and I invented this mathematical fantasy. In this fantasy, we used a new currency, we called it "EV", to buy luck. "EV" is short for "expected value", which is defined mathematically as what you might expect to get out of random events if you were paid for specific outcomes. For example, if you decided to gamble with coin flips, and you paid one dollar for every flip, but you won two dollars for times the coin ended on heads, you would expect to break even. It is possible that you might lose money after a certain number of coin flips, but you might make money, too. I claimed that my lifetime results based on all "random" events were well below expected value, and the doctor in Ann Arbor provided evidence and justification for my grumbling. Josh's mathematical skill and wit turned this into something fun and beautiful. "You're just saving up EV, Dad," he told me. "Now you can cash in by having a better-than-expected outcome with your treatments!"

We both know that probability does not care about past events. Neither of us truly believe that "luck" is really a thing. But his idea was enough to teach me to shrug off bad breaks in life. For example, if I missed a long putt in golf by an inch to the left, but then a wind swings by and rolls the ball off the green into the sand, then I was really just putting EV into my "luck" bank account to be cashed in later. It does not really work that way, but I wish I had used that as a coping mechanism for when things inexplicably went badly throughout the earlier years of my life.

This line of faulty reasoning, this game that we played to deal with being dealt a bad hand, seemed to make sense when my response to treatments kept me reasonably healthy for much longer than expected. I started to embrace past "bad luck" episodes, like when I suffered through a flat tire on the turnpike into Chicago during rush hour, or when my phone started ringing as wrapped up my sermon as a guest preacher at a large church, or when my long awaited camping trip was washed out with oceans of rain in spite of our careful planning based on the forecast's "near zero" chance of precipitation. I was simply saving EV.

*****

Hope, of course, is more than numbers. In its grandest sense, it is a longing for our loftiest reality, a life-defining orientation based on what we treasure most deeply, and how we dream the best of all futures. It represents an ideal that is not yet fully ours. My consideration of which treatment options provided the strongest *medical* hope ran parallel with my fixation on this *other*, this *grandest* hope. If there is ever a time my faith was to have relevance for my own life, it was here. I cannot say that as my chances of survival faded, my hope in the afterlife grew stronger. But I did spend more time thinking about it.

Most of my thinking was pure speculation. Nobody really knows what our experience is after death, what it looks like, what it feels like, what it smells like, or what it sounds like; or if there are any senses at all. But to console and humor myself, I would play mind games, pondering what it would be like to chat with Johann Sebastian at one of the Bach family reunions, or to quaff a stein with Martin Luther to see what he was really like, or to interview Alex Trebek to get responses in the form of questions. Maybe nothing is trivial there, even with him.

Hope as a piece of the Christian faith sprouts up from Scripture. The Bible explores various sides of hope ranging from hope as national political aspirations, to longing for the afterlife, to hope as a general virtue. Some have concluded that our final hope is a promise from God that diminishes the physical limitations of this life. But I would not blame someone suffering from cancer to see a hope in the afterlife as cashing in a warranty for a defective product. Whichever facet of that glimmering diamond is shining in those ancient texts, it is certainly not a mathematical concept. Instead, whether used in a collective sense for a group of people or a personal attribute, almost all uses of "hope" in the Bible have a strong emotional component.

Without getting into too many details, I will highlight two examples that became very important to me in my cancer experience. In one of the earliest books of the New Testament, the Apostle Paul wants to teach his audience about what happens to their loved ones when they die, "So that you don't grieve as other people do who do not have hope." (1 Thessalonians 4:14). While this letter of Paul's describes parts of the experience beyond the grave, what struck me squarely in the heart was the contrast between *grieving* and *having hope*. In any context, having hope seems to be a powerful antidote to crippling grief that is too often part of life.

As treatments started to prove an effective combatant against my cancerous enemies, I realized and embraced more fully the emotional side of hope. While numbers always remained important for me in making treatment decisions, Hope became an ally in a war where one cannot have too many friends.

The other piece of holy writ that I held close to my heart is from Jeremiah, the so-called "Weeping Prophet". His nickname is well deserved. Driven by the compassion he had for his nation, he cried, "O that my head were a spring of water, and my eyes a fountain of tears, so that I might weep day and night for the slain of my poor people!" (Jeremiah 9:1, *NRSV*) His grief resonates with mine when I look at the senseless hatred humanity wreaks upon itself.

But even in his grief, he talks about hope. Speaking on behalf of his God, he proclaims, "For surely I know the plans I have for you, says the LORD, plans for your welfare and not for harm, to give you a future with hope. (Jeremiah 29:11, *NRSV*) What struck me then and continues to impress me now is how hope is a future concept. It would be demoralizing had he talked about "a future that sucks as badly as your current condition."

Hope is a cheerful attitude about a future that we want to enter. As much as I wanted to survive just one more day, all my imagined scenes were of a beautiful experience surrounded by love and joy and peace and comfort. Whether I lived or died, that is how the future looked to me; so, either way, hope is a win.

6 SURVIVING

Nobody ever won a game by resigning
– Attributed to Savielly Tartakower, Grandmaster of Chess

It was the day before Thanksgiving and we had just gotten off the phone with my Aunt Cheryl, finalizing plans for our family feast. We had a long tradition of celebrating Thanksgiving at my parents' house because it was Mom's way to share her world-class food artistry with our extended family. Indeed, her food was why the word "sumptuous" was invented. However, in recent years, especially since Dad died, Jenn and I offered to host the celebration. It was a logical move since Mom's family mostly lived in Michigan. Besides, Aunt Cheryl, who shared a special sister bond with Mom, always welcomed her for an extended visit for the days surrounding the holiday.

But this year, shortly after arriving at Cheryl's, Mom suffered a stroke. Plans for Thanksgiving were scrapped, of course, but our Wednesday morning phone call centered around details of visiting Mom in the hospital while trying to salvage what remained of a celebration. Jenn and I lay in bed pondering why this awful thing had to happen during the season that defined so much about who she was. But we'll get through this, we thought. She had survived a mild stroke before, and we did not really know how bad this one was.

It was then that I complained of an acute pain shooting up from behind my navel into the left side of my neck. This was surely not worth worrying about; I had survived chemo, weight loss that shoved me to the precipice of death, and radiation therapy earlier that year. I was merely being attacked on the inside by some beans, angry from my feeble attempts to digest its roughage. But, ugh, the pain was horrible. Maybe it was a heart attack, but I recalled the scene in "Norma Rae" when Vernon's heart attack was first indicated by a numbness in his left arm, and my left arm was normal. But I suppose they do not give board certifications to practice medicine based on what you learn from cinema, so what do I know?

Shoving past my objections, Jenn called 911 and asked for an ambulance to transport me to the hospital. The person handling the call suggested this might be a heart attack and advised me to slowly chew on a single aspirin while the ambulance rushed to our house. By the time the vehicle arrived, most of the pain had subsided so I really thought I could by-pass the gurney and all that. Besides really despising people making a big deal out of anything about me, I really, really hated being considered unable to transport myself. By way of compromise, they allowed me to walk down the stairs but strapped me onto the gurney, anyway. Then they rolled me to the ambulance. I was in reasonably good spirits, and besides, this was a new experience. I'll treat this like a ride at Disney World, but less fun and incredibly, almost as expensive.

Once at the hospital, I felt good enough to be embarrassed that I was wasting all their precious time and space. While COVID quarantine was still largely in effect, patient rooms were in very short supply, and many of my fellow recipients of emergency attention were scattered along the edges of the hallway. Yet, heart attack continued to be the prime suspect prompting doctors and nurses to hook wires, tubes, electrodes, and whatever else to guard me against death from cardiac failure.

Though I thought the pain had left completely, it was merely catching its breath so it could charge with dominating furor. A few years prior to this, my right ureter, the tube that connects the kidney to the urinary bladder, played host to a half-pea sized stone. I read then that a kidney stone could be the closest pain a male is likely ever to experience on par with childbirth. I'm pretty sure that this latter experience was worse.

When I had time to catch my breath enough to engage my brain, I played mind games asking whether I would be willing to go through an hour of this torment if I could stave off cancer indefinitely. Further, would I agree to suffer through this much daily as the extortion cancer demanded? I answered that I would. It was here that I realized that it was not pain that I was afraid of. Nor did I tremble as Death waited nearby. It was the invasion of a cruel parasite, a cellular collective that thrives on the health of my good cells, colonizing other tissues throughout my body. Yes, that's it! Cancer is the uninvited interloper that steals health, plans, families, and life.

When Socrates was preparing to drink the hemlock that would kill him, his students and friends wept miserably, presumably for his sake. But he urged them not to fear death, because who really knows what is on the other side? And why should we fear what will certainly be better for us? The Apostle Paul was even less unsure than Socrates when he affirmed that dying is gain. I'm not saying that I was looking forward to death even though I could affirm God's great post-life party. But for me, it was not so much entering that place afterwards, whatever it is like, as it was the fact that you cannot turn back. If it was only anticipating what lies ahead, I would, like Tim Keller, look forward to meeting my sweet Jesus. Honestly, I have never been afraid of death. I just did not want to leave Jenn and Caleb.

However, cancer's intrusiveness is what I hate most. Cancer is not just an illness; it is an invasion of everything that represents life. Maybe my hatred of its invasion stems from our family's Florida vacation in my teenage years. My folks did not make a bunch of money, but they managed it well, at least most of the time. And I worked at a job I loathed to save up some extra money for fun stuff. So, harnessing our inner-Griswold, we loaded up our car and headed to the land of Sunshine and Citrus. This may have been our first trip where housing accommodations were via motels. So, upon arrival at the inn next to the beach, we excitedly planted our stuff in our room and tore off to the ocean.

One of the most glaring exceptions to our family's good money management occurred as we were leaving town. In those days, credit cards were not universally accepted, so we normally would buy a vacation's worth of traveler's checks for the trip's transactions. Before leaving for Florida, however, both Mom and Dad had worked late enough that the banks were all closed, and we left home with the least secure bartering tender ever: cash. I had my summer's savings, earned through sweaty, greasy toil, and my folks had their vacation account money. Our excitement to get to the beach was enough of an invitation for some well-known crime team to extract all of our funds from our vulnerable motel room.

I'm not sure what upset me more, the early termination of our vacation, or the evaporation of the fruit of hundreds of hours of honest work. But I am certain that the central agony in all of this, the thing that annoyed me the most and for the longest time was how someone else invaded our sacred space without a care to the suffering they caused us. That is you, Cancer, you cursed wretch!

*****

I have never been a good runner, but I always embraced a challenge. So, when my friend Monty invited me to a 5K run in the little town of Darlington, Indiana, I eagerly accepted. Although I was a miler in my earlier years, I had never run that far while being timed, and certainly I had never run that far in competition. But to authentically pursue this challenge, I laid out a strict training regimen of eating whatever I wanted and burning it off with practice runs. I'm proud of the fact that I met my training goals: The former piece (eating whatever I wanted) very consistently, and the latter piece (practice runs) once. In my defense, physical conditioning was something I always did with a ball sport when you kept score. I was less motivated by health or athletic factors than my disgust of losing a game.

That motivation was enough to bring me to Darlington's starting line surrounded by a gaggle of athletes that strikingly resembled those marathoners I had seen during the Olympics. Therefore, I was motivated by a trio of factors: The challenge of a competition (it wasn't really a competition), the world class caliber of my opponents (they were neither opponents nor world class), and the fear of embarrassing myself (nobody else cared how I finished). Being in decent shape for a non-runner but having no idea how far five kilometers is in terms of pacing, I broke out of the gates, quite proud that I was giving these famous Olympians (they weren't) a run for their money. Just as I started to feel the joy of completing the run—and just in time because I was completely spent—I saw a sign indicating that I was approaching the half-way mark. Reality bites hard sometimes. Honestly, I was on the precipice of expelling everything I had consumed that morning, but I reminded myself that I am not a quitter. Somehow, I kept going.

Over the next burning mile or so, the urge to hurl subsided and I reached a slower, more reasonable pace. Shortly, I heard crowds cheering as some of the premier runners blasted down the final stretch. The route in Darlington began in the town's main street, spent a longish portion winding through a neighborhood, then re-entered the main street for the spectator-lined homestretch, so I reasoned that the end was near. I said I had been a miler in my early years, and my only virtue as a middle-distance runner then, other than the ability to tolerate misery, was my better than average final kick. I reasoned that if I could make it out to the main drag soon, I could finish with a strong kick and avoid bringing shame to my family and to my country.

My strength, bolstered by the cheers of the crowd, returned as I switched on my jets. I was sure I could finish this last eighth of a mile or so with something that resembled a sprint. So, I ignored pain, ignored shortage of oxygen, and pursued the finish line like a pro. The problem was that I did not see the finish line. Where is the finish line? I've surely been on Main Street long enough, right? The whole population of Darlington could not have filled more than a couple hundred yards, but as I looked up, I could only see a mass of cheering people leading up to the vanishing point. The finish line was purely a theory. I assured myself that it was there, wherever "there" was, and kept running. I realized that it is impossible to slow your sprint when crowds are cheering.

I have thought about that experience many times in the years since. I have known since eighth grade when I was almost lapped in a track meet that I was not a good runner, and I could only win races if I put slow enough people around me. However, there may be two things I possess in abundance: Stubbornness and pain tolerance. Those two attributes rose to prominence in my life that day.

It still amazes me how different the pain bearing experience feels when you really do not know when the suffering will end. Finishing a task or going through tough times are different—maybe easier—when we know when it will end. But when the end is literally not in sight, when the finish line to suffering disappears into the vanishing point, we are subjected to a completely different experience. There must be something about the way we are stingy about what remains in our tolerance tank when we do not know when we are completely depleted. Knowing where the end is, though, sometimes allows us to find inner resources from beyond ourselves for just one more hit.

But it was not any level of pain tolerance that brought me to the finish line in Darlington. It was my other trait, rarely classified as a virtue: My stubbornness. Little did I know how stubbornness would play a role years later on the eve of Thanksgiving.

*****

After treating my phantom heart attack, the ER staff asked if I was able to sit. I said I could. So, they placed me in a reclining chair that would have fit in someone's den; that is, if it had not been so intolerably uncomfortable with bile-green upholstery. But that is fine since I was apparently in better shape than the other poor souls who lined the hospital's hall. Once every thirty minutes or so, a nurse scampered by to check on my status which, for the first couple hours, was manageable. But have you ever regretted telling a waiter that you did not need a coffee refill because you did not realize they were asking, "Will you ever, in your life, need a refill?" It is a very different question.

Then, without so much as a whisper suggesting a return to action, the pain that began my morning struck with vengeance. Within minutes, my voice involuntarily howled with enough force to echo in the halls, but apparently not enough volume to get anyone's attention. I do not know how I managed it, but I looked ahead at other patients and hoped their issues were not severe. My situation, after all, was surely temporary. Pain is temporary, after all; victory lasts forever. Pain is temporary, after all, but I'll get through this thing. Pain is temporary, after all, but putting up with it and getting through it is what I do. These and countless other misleading and unhelpful truths raced through my mind as I continued to howl.

A few times over the next couple hours, nurses would swing by. This time, though, they were not checking on how good I felt; my groans made that obvious. They simply wanted to tell me that they were short on doctors, and they were going to get to me as quickly as possible. "Can you give me something for my pain?" I pleaded.

Her sympathetic "I'll see what the doctor says" would serve as her farewell for a long, long, long, long time. It is amazing to me how our perception of time often has nothing to do with the number of seconds ticking past.

My thoughts careened in all directions. "If there's time for the doctor to assess the appropriate medication, why can't she see me?" I demanded internally. "Just gimme *anything!*" The wonders of a stressed mind to think only absurdities while leaving them unuttered remains my only shining star of that moment.

Eventually, they administered some minor league drug that lowered the pain's volume from 11 to 10. I'm still screaming, but there was a strange satisfaction in knowing the doctor did not lose track of me. And finally, she arrived with a grim look on her face. "You have a hole in your stomach."

Again, words constructed in my head did not materialize in my mouth: So what? There's no reason to look like someone died.

Her continuation justified her fatal expression. They could operate, she explained, but I would have only a 50-50 chance of survival. On the other hand, we can leave it alone and maybe it will heal up on its own. They informed me that it would be a long process, and an uncomfortable one.

My brain again silently argued. "Who knows? That passive approach may work. And who knows? Maybe unicorns will also come in and save me. It does not sound like much of a plan of action." Either way, I calculated about an even chance of survival. Put another way, that meant that I had about an even chance of *not* surviving. Dying or living for me was now a coin flip.

If it is a coin flip, I at least have the privilege of choosing the coin. For me, it was an easy choice. I recalled a few years earlier when Jeff, my younger brother, had surgery to fix an umbilical hernia. Somehow, the surgeon nicked a bowel and sent Jeff into a coma that lasted two weeks. He survived, but barely. So, I decided to flip the coin that would at least allow me to be aware of the fight for survival. Surgery then became the passive choice. If I tried to let the hole in my stomach close on its own, I would at least be aware of the fight. I wanted awareness and I wanted a battle. My confidence surged. I wanted pain and injuries and death to cower before my stubbornness!

Jenn later told me many of the details that I did not know or could not process at the time. When the emergency room doctor estimated even odds with the surgical option, she had not yet read my history of targeted radiation therapy. They determined that the hole was probably caused by the stomach tissue's weakening from that therapy. The staff became certain that my odds became closer to flipping a coin and hoping it would land on the edge. Survival of my chosen plan was roughly the same.

Another conversation that floated above my awareness was the doctor telling Jenn that they would do their best to keep me alive long enough for my children to come say good-bye. My experience of pain blotted out that whole conversation even though I was right there when it happened. So, seeing Rachel and Josh puzzled me at the time, but makes a lot of sense in light of the importance of final farewells.

I have never been one to give up. When Jim Valvano announced the V Foundation for Cancer Research shortly before he died, he declared its motto, "Don't give up . . . don't ever give up." It is hard not to be inspired by his life, his foundation, and his motto. But not giving up is more than simply not resigning. You can also give up by failing to put your complete effort into prevailing. Often, most often, maybe, surviving requires fighting, holding nothing back to give yourself the best chance.

After three days, receiving confirmation that the hole in my stomach had completely closed, I *walked* out of the hospital. The doctors caring for me told me I was a miracle.

7 PLAYING

Play is a preparation for religious life, and one of the chief
means of its realization.
– Carl E. Seashore, 1910

My father was a loving, honest man. As a child of the depression,
the other pieces of his virtue were largely filled in by the prevailing
ethics of his childhood: God, country, and responsibility. While he
could play and have fun, these more serious traits dominated his
outlook on life.

Therefore, maybe it was a form of rebellion that prompted me to
view "playing" as a virtue. Maybe it was my creativity to add to the
traditional lists of *Heavenly Virtues* the need to play. Or maybe it
was just my own lack of seriousness in Dad's stern sense of
rightness that carved out space for playing as part of everyday life.
Whatever it was, the need to play was enough motivation to get
out of bed and continue my life.

In pre-adolescence one of my favorite things to do was to field fly
balls that my dad would knock out to me. Having mastered simple
popups at an early age, I loved those that were far enough out of
reach that a diving catch was required. (It is no surprise that the
dive catch experience infected Caleb.)

The problem with my extreme love of such baseball activities was that my willing partner—in this case, Dad—could only last for about fifteen minutes. However, I theorize that I could've kept fielding his flies for several hours, a theory I was never able to test. After a quarter hour stretch of almost physical activity, his standard phrase to release him of the burden of play was, "I need a breather. I'm too old for this!"

The irony that I detected even then, at the tender age of ten, was that his breather involved squatting in our backyard and lighting up a cigarette. Even then, in the mid-1960s, evidence was sufficient to inform us of the lack of wisdom associated with smoking tobacco. Even then, I estimated that a serious God-centered, country-loving responsible adult could last at least an hour if he did not smoke. What was more in rhythm of the times was that Dad's mid-thirty age was enough to call him an aging man. I remember an episode of "Gomer Pyle, USMC" centering around Sergeant Carter's thirty-fifth birthday, and the humor cascading from the commonly accepted notion that, yeah, that's getting old.

But that blend of irony and unacceptable assessment about aging prompted a commitment—even then—that I would never, ever let age itself stop me from having fun by being active. I know other situations in life can force a person to stop doing what they love the most, but there would always be some healthy activity that I would do as long as I had health, and I committed to doing my best to assure I could maintain most of my body parts' functionality.

But reality can rip through the sturdiest plans without breaking a sweat. Decades later, in the throes of debilitating side effects from chemotherapy, my biggest challenges did not involve balls and bats and gloves, but forks and plates and stairs and toothbrushes. My desire to get out and play again was mostly thwarted by the very physical inability I vowed to stave off from childhood.

A few weeks before my strength was completely decimated, I did manage to get into a game. Jenn's circle of tennis friends had taken up pickleball and we received an invitation to go watch. "You could play, too, Jenn," I insisted. "I love to watch you play!"

But at my normal activity level, sports and games are not for watching, they are for participating. While Jenn and her friends were slapping the noisy, plastic ball back and forth, I was silently hoping for an invitation. But I was also silently afraid of an invitation, because on this chilly, early spring day, my quadriceps, which had once filled the upper legs of my pants too broad for my waist, were emaciated and thinner by far than my knees. All of this sickliness was hidden by my warmup pants that flapped against my femur dominated upper legs. Besides issues of vanity, I did not know how I could possibly move enough or stay upright sufficiently to play a competitive sport.

The other challenge, of course, was that I had never learned the mysterious art of turning down an invitation to participate in a sporting event. So, I found myself playing pickleball, a sport that I had previously regarded as a gateway drug to checkers and euchre.

Alright, I will not insult the sport. Indeed, the women I played with that day were pretty good and had no problem at all showing me how athletic pickleball could be, and how unathletic I was at the time. Jane, a supreme athlete and competitor—while simultaneously exhibiting the most perfect gracious generosity—hit a stinging shot to my backhand, which I tried to put back into play. Unfortunately, when I planted my right foot to return the ball, my leg crumbled beneath me and I skittered across the surface of an adjoining court.

Of course, everyone wanted to make sure I was still in one piece, which I mostly was, physically, except the smear of blood and skin I painted on the pavement behind me. My low platelet count revealed some minor problems in trying to heal my already prominent knee. Worse, the fallout at being unable to catch myself, even in my degraded state, served up emotional trauma I chewed on for weeks.

By and by, I started seeing my scrapes and bruises in a positive light. Would anyone else get out there to play such brutal pickleball in the state I was in? Would anyone else lay it all out there, risking life and limb, when it really might be life or limb, for something as gladiatorial as pickleball? I think not!

*****

I once heard someone say that sports are a microcosm of life. In other words, you can learn a lot about life from sports because sports are a miniature form of life. There is competition, there are winners, there are losers, there is abuse, there is frustration, everything is expensive, and there is occasionally—but not always—reward for effort and dignity. Through sports we also learn how to cooperate, how to live within rules that some non-playing legislators foist upon us, and how to accept the usual—but not always—authoritative judgment of someone else. Indeed, to learn sports well is to learn most there is to know about life.

It is not that life and sports are the same thing. The high school basketball coach I admired most when I was a young man suffered a fatal heart attack at halftime in one of his teams' games. His last words were, "OK, boys, let's play basketball!" But basketball was not his life. Sports were not a body of obsessions that he needed in order to find meaning in life. Rather, he was an earnest, heroic man who loved his family, the guys on his teams, and his God, and made everyone around him a better person. Basketball was simply one way he chose to express his full participation in the beauty of life.

What would it be like to live your life completely until the very end, to participate in that one thing above all others that gets you out of bed in the morning, that thing for which you have such passion that other concerns of life fall into a distant second place? I always wondered about that and wondered about whether I would carry my passion for living to the very end. Or would I, like so many others, run out of enthusiasm and run out of energy and just lie down, bored. I have often wondered what kind of thinking about life would encourage me to fall into such a dispassionate state that I no longer had that one thing. It was with this sentiment, I vowed I would not face the emaciation of chemo lying down, literally, as long as I had strength to stand.

*****

Aging is an endless flow of compromise. In my mid-thirties, my orthopedic surgeon advised me to stop playing basketball, advice which I was happy to ignore. Yet, from that point endlessly into the future, I could not deny the ever-expanding catalog of activities that I would either give up or continue playing with pain and a drop in performance, and the expanding inventory of physical problems that fed into that catalog.

But this was a reality for which I mapped out a plan since high school. Left knee surgery in eleventh grade with the promise of lifelong challenges on that side prompted me to find other avenues of passion. Thus, I fell in love with chess.

My early love affair with the "royal game" is as unusual as it is steamy. In its heyday in my life, my passion for the game knew no bounds. My abandonment of reason and prudence scales to other visceral love interests like Romeo's love for Juliet or the biblical Samson's passion for almost anyone. I once confessed in college that I would rather spend my Friday nights playing chess than on a date with anyone, a statement fueled by a recent breakup. Chess would never do *that* to me!

I now know that my passion for chess in early adulthood was more of an infatuation than a true lifelong romantic commitment. I saw early on that without a more robust set of intellectual tools and a more sedentary physical inclination, chess would never be for me the primary road to eternal happiness others have found it to be. Bobby Fischer, who won the world chess championship in 1972, famously declared, "All I want to do, ever, is play chess." I could never subscribe to a game as the true path to Nirvana, but I did decide to keep a spectator's interest in my hip pocket in case other activities abandoned me.

I do not regret giving up competitive chess; I was not good enough to win often and I do not often enjoy losing. So, I follow the sport as a spectator with enough interest to care about tournament outcomes and enough understanding to know what is going on. But perhaps my most important fringe benefit from chess has been an understanding about myself, and what it takes to keep me engaged in an activity. I suggested above that my inherent gifts as a chess player were not extensive. I was not horrible, though, and I did not mind spending long hours trying to understand the game as deeply as I could.

Besides, I have always had the need to do something. Maybe my childhood pleas for something to do, when answered by my mom's stereotypical parental reply, "You could clean your room," were not specific enough. What I should have said during those long—too long, in fact—summer vacations was, "I need something to do that is challenging, something that will allow me to express myself creatively, something that offers an enjoyable growth path, and something that I'm passionate about. And cleaning my room does not qualify." Of course I would still have to clean my room, but then I could go looking for the challenge, creativity, growth, and passion elsewhere.

*****

The main thing that chess does not quench is the itch to move my body. When we migrated back to Michigan after my initial cancer diagnosis, fate decreed that we would live about a mile from a local golf course whose membership fit into our budget. Since I needed something to get me out of the house, and since my frugality would force me to do so whenever possible to get the most value from the membership fee, I found myself on the golf course almost every day, regardless of the weather; or, as Jenn reminded me, regardless of my inability to stand up on my own two legs.

My strength was zapped and my normal daily dose of tennis or softball or volleyball was out of the question. Though golf was never something I lived to do and I was never that good at it, it was a fair compromise while hindered by chemo induced weakness. It satisfied my need to get outside and swing at *something*. Even in the latter days of my chemotherapy treatments when rising from bed became a hideous challenge, the wet, chilly days of central Michigan in April were beckoning me to arise, go forth, and hit something outside.

On a good day with perfect health, golf has always been the four-letter-noun that tests my soul. But then, even the mixture of golf's inherent frustration with the wraith-like physical stature that remained after chemo, was not enough to extinguish the itch to get outside and do something.

Yet, after my first few treatments of chemo, a CT scan revealed a blood clot in my lungs which required hammering my body with additional drugs to thin my blood and dissipate the clot. One side effect was that the new medicine also thinned out other fluids in my body, including the stuff that is supposed to stay in my sinuses. My nose was a leaky faucet I could not shut off, and this new development was just another way in which my formerly athletic body was betraying me. Still, I needed to get out and play.

Some around me thought my frequent visitation with the golf course was some kind of obsession. In my weakened, leaky faucet state, I was unable to hit the ball a respectable distance. At times, what I was doing would not meet the definition of "fun" found in anyone's dictionary. Yet, I maintain that golf was not an obsession for me. And later, when I was able, other activities were not obsessions even though my impaired physical condition continued to add frustration to my activities and forced me to vastly lower my performance expectations.

Indeed, my need to go out and play was not an obsession, but a demonstration that I was still alive. It also stopped being about improving a skill, a concept that I had nurtured in my psyche for most of my life. As I said earlier, I always regarded my previous days of life as preparation for the next thing. That applies to playing, too. Every time I played, I wanted to learn as much as possible so that next time, I would be better prepared. But when the future is in doubt, improvement as a primary goal is scattered into the wind and becomes less important. So, why did I play? Playing was a way to remove myself from the bed I thought I was going to die on; to continue embracing life as something that is lived actively rather than succumbing to sickness and death as masters of my being. Rather than improving at a game, going out to golf, however weakly, was my way of defeating cancer. Lew: 1, Cancer: 0.

It did not matter how I felt or how I played or what the weather was like that spring; I always played a full round of 18 holes, issuing a pocket veto to Jenn's suggestion to take care of my body and only play a sensible nine holes. It may not have been the wisest series of decisions I have made, but these hours on the golf course by myself—I almost always played by myself—offered solace and therapy for my spirit. Plus, I cashed in on the ample opportunities to explore the philosophical side of life, of golf, and the huge areas where the two intersected. To wit: Why am I golfing when it is likely that I will be dead before the golf season is over? Should I try to become a better golfer? Why? So that I can carry these newfound skills with me to the grave? For that matter, why should anyone golf? Perhaps I am golfing as a way to disrespect cancer's attempts to control my life. Or maybe I golf because it is the only way to satisfy my lifelong obsession—planted in those early days with my father in the backyard catching fly balls—to be moving, doing *something*, while there is still daylight.

Or maybe my engagement with golf was my entry to get back to normal, the beginning of healing even if I did not know how well my treatments were working. In fact, the effectiveness of chemo and the later radiation did not determine whether I could play. As my weight continued to plummet, I was certainly going to play because playing, for me, is virtue, and it is life.

8 COMPLAINING

> "The air of the country is sharp, the rocks many, the trees innumerable, the grass little, the winter cold, the summer hot, the gnats in summer biting, the wolves at midnight howling, etc."
> – *The History of the Colony of Massachusets-Bay*, quoted by Thomas Hutchinson, 1764

Mr. Henry always greeted me with a warm smile when I saw him at church. Although he was over a half century older, I would always look for him before the Sunday morning music started. He always reminded me how good God is and how blessed he feels to have lived through so much for so long. His old age was punctuated by long outmoded polyester sports coats and huge prescription glasses that added a touch of gravity to his cheerful expression. Mrs. Henry, always by his side, never said anything other than our customary greeting in a weak voice befitting of her frail and wizened stature.

I learned that Mr. Henry had been diagnosed with some type of bone cancer that may have gone unnoticed until his femur snapped when he was getting out of bed. My concern for my aged friend prompted me to visit him in the hospital. When I learned that his prognosis was grim, I expected to see an old friend who was in shock, in pain, and in denial. What I found, though, was a man furious at the incompetence of everyone around him, and angry with everything and everyone within reach. "Why didn't these doctors see this cancer earlier? Why can't they give me something for the pain? Why does it have to be cancer? Why are these beds so damned uncomfortable? Why can't they offer me a blanket or something? Why do the lights flicker so much?" Then, toward me, "Why are you here, anyway?"

I meekly offered, "Do you want to pray?"

"Go ahead," he said. "Then leave!"

I was surprised by Mr. Henry's display of furor, but I understood. If there was ever a time to criticize circumstances or people or God, even if nobody is at fault, that would be the time. Besides, being told there is nothing anyone can do to keep you alive, that prospect of dying, or pain so intense that you wish you could, tinkers with your emotions.

I never saw Mr. Henry again. I was advised not to burden him with a return visit, a request I heartily embraced.

He died a few days after my visit with him. I wondered what his final hours were like, whether he was in pain, or even aware as his heartbeats and breaths finally stopped. But even more, I wondered about Mrs. Henry, and if her unassuming, laconic presence had also been singed by her spouse's angry reaction to his plight.

*****

I had often thought about Mr. Henry, his life, his suffering, and his death, and how I might have responded to having my joyous existence torpedoed by such an awful thing as cancer. I wondered if it was possible for anyone in that situation to rise above the circumstances and keep their sense of joy or manners in much the same way they seemed to throughout their normal course of living.

I used to think I could do it. I embraced the myth that my attitude in any situation is something I have complete control over. Good feelings can simply be produced through the "mind over matter" formula, and if cheer in the face of death and suffering has any benefit at all, then I can die with a smile on my face.

I also used to think of my own death in terms similar to the painful deaths of martyrs throughout history. Saint Lawrence, according to fanciful legend, was being grilled—literally—for his faith by Emperor Valerian. But he did not complain that his life was roasting away. Rather, he simply joked that, "you can turn me over now; I'm done on this side."

Maybe I take my life and aversion to pain too seriously. Maybe Mr. Henry did, too. But the big difference is that Saint Lawrence, according to this tradition, died for some cause. Whether or not he was accomplishing anything through his dying, there was a cause that motivated the emperor to extinguish him, and it was that cause that he regarded more highly than his life or than avoidance of torture.

But cancer is a pointless enemy. We might suffer, bleed, and die to cancer, but there is no redemption and no salvation. Our loss is a total loss, and there is no beneficiary for our martyrdom.

I think I understand the complaints of the cancer patient. Even before my own pointless misery, I had deep compassion for Mr. Henry and I understood, in a second-hand way, why he might have complained so deeply during his suffering. Even before my diagnosis, I discovered that my complaining threshold is much lower, and my capacity to criticize reality much higher when I am in pain or other forms of discomfort. "Mind over matter" is much more difficult to achieve when my mind is distracted with suffering, pain, and imminent death.

*****

In George Bernard Shaw's five-part play, "Back to Methuselah", the serpent pontificates in her conversation with Eve (Shaw identifies the serpent as a female), "You see things; and you say 'Why?' But I dream things that never were; and I say 'Why not?'" These words were repeated by John F. Kennedy in 1963 as he addressed the Irish Parliament, and again by Robert Kennedy in a slightly altered form while campaigning in 1968, and again by Edward Kennedy at Robert's funeral. If I understand the spirit of the age in the 1960s, America was consumed with dreaming and imagining possibilities, especially since many of its citizens perceived the race with its cold war adversary as being a tight, life-and-death contest. This competitive spirit rang true whether it was a space race, an arms race, or playing a game of theoretical political dominoes. I must admit, hearing John Kennedy's speech, and Robert Kennedy's slightly different rendition seem to be a bit inspiring. It launches my imagination into thinking what could be done to promote good in the world and rid it of so much evil, although the quote represents the words of humanity's arch-villain in reptilian form.

The main point of the use of Shaw's line in the president's speech in Dublin in 1963 was to move us beyond settling for reality as it is and complaining about it, and dreaming of a reality that we do not have, and working toward it. The former attitude is represented by my own personal least favorite cliches in modern parlance, namely, "It is what it is." As I mentioned, the rebuttal is simply asserting that "It isn't what isn't!" Of course, neither line makes any sense because they both make perfect sense, being always true.

But in broad strokes, the serpent's line (ironically delivered in the paradise of the garden of Eden where the status quo really ought to be pretty good), and the Kennedys' use of it are soft forms of complaint about a reality that we might be able to change. Perhaps there is something ennobling about envisioning a future in which a well implemented plan makes things better for the common good. It sounds great, doesn't it?

The problem with cancer—and some forms more than others—is that there is often very little the sufferer can do about it. I mentioned earlier that I had given up asking the why questions, and in my conversations with my oncologist and other knowledgeable specialists, I learned the futility of most of my "why not?" suggestions.

But as long as treatments were presented to me as a way of stemming the progression of my bodily tissues' interlopers, I was willing to take them. And as I was taking these amazingly complicated and astronomically expensive treatments, my list of problems stemming from the treatments to keep me alive continued to grow. And as this list of problems continued to grow, I found myself less focused on gratitude that I'm surviving well beyond anyone's expectation, and more aware of the needling little foibles of post-treatment life. It was then that I realized that I complain too much.

Maybe the part of my experience that I'm most embarrassed about, or maybe a little bit (or a lot) ashamed about is that I eventually became accustomed to survival months beyond statistical averages. At various points, I was able to return to doing things I had done all my life, like volleyball, bicycling, and tennis, although not with the strength or balance or timing that had once been well tuned. Even playing tennis and even understanding that I would have to consciously lower my performance expectations by a wide margin, just being *out there, playing*, should have been enough to bring tears of happiness rolling down my cheeks. Instead, I would often complain that I'm too slow and too inept and ridiculous in every conceivable athletic way, and that tennis is a stupid game. At least the way that I play it. It was not always my cry, but it was a complaint I voiced tragically too often.

*****

But I do not think I'm the only person who complains too much.

A couple years before my diagnosis, I was working my way through the scarce pre-dawn December light from my bus stop to my downtown office. The journey was pleasant this morning because the wind was calm, the snow had stopped, and the temperature was a warmish twenty degrees. Yet, I am not one to dawdle when a destination lies ahead, so I looked for diagonals from sidewalk to sidewalk, crisscrossing the empty streets with beautiful efficiency.

At one point, I took note of an old van lumbering toward me at a breakneck speed of twenty miles per hour or so. There was no danger, but I scampered across the street so I did not cause the driver any alarm. My safety precautions were not enough of a buffer to prevent the driver from stopping in the middle of the avenue, complaining: "You need to get a reflective coat if you're gonna' walk downtown before daylight! I could barely see you!"

I was so surprised by this infusion of advice from a stranger that I did not have time to remember that my coat was, indeed, reflective. But what I did fully appreciate was the fact that this stranger, in all of her ambition to register a complaint, had forgotten to turn her headlights on. My coat did not function as a reflective coat because there was no light to reflect. "Um, excuse me," I began, "but your headlights aren't on."

With that, she rolled up her window and sped away. I enjoyed the rest of my morning and had great fun sharing my experience with others in the office, as we pondered the human capacity to complain. We speculated what it would have been like for the driver to get home, and would she still complain about my jaywalking incompetence, or would she swallow her complaint and—against all odds and against normal human behavior—learn that complaining is not always justified.

*****

Some things are actually worth complaining about, even if our complaints don't get us very far. When I was about eight years old, my family went to a small, local fair. The kind with rides and cotton candy, and games rigged so that even winners take home prizes worth less than the cost to play. I had somehow gotten permission and the required quarter to play one of those games where you turn this crank that operates a crane that will grab a prize and drop it into a chute. My young eyes were fascinated by that device. I mean, what could be easier? And those prizes are all so glittery! Probably real gold, eh?

I remember transferring my gifted twenty-five cents from my sweaty palm to the woman behind the counter, remembering her now as one with all the sweetness and maternal kindness as Gunnery Sergeant Hartman in the movie "Full Metal Jacket". I nervously started to turn the crank, and quickly, I clutched a toy in the jaws of this crane and maneuvered it around to the chute. It was ready to drop when the gunnery sergeant stomped by and grabbed my toy, put it back into the pile, and told me to go away.

Who does that to little kids? Maybe this gave me perspective, but I always hated fairs for the rest of my life. Was this the wakeup call that I needed to teach me that this world with all its people, with all its chaos, is not Utopia? Or was this purely a positive experience, and I can now say, with Joseph and his technicolor Dreamcoat, "She meant to hurt this little kid, but God used it to teach me about life!" Or maybe the tears of sorrow often water the seeds of life's important lessons.

There are so many other pieces of reality that most people I know freely complain about. Many of these pieces are things that will probably never change. And so, we could accept the meanness of people and placidly go about our lives. Or maybe we just become more selective with what we're willing to spend the energy to complain about.

Just because humans have not learned to harness the power of one of our most practiced skills, complaining, that has not hindered our efforts to perfect it. Complaining fills in that huge gap between life as we know it and life as we want it to be. It replaces the pointless resignation of the loathsome, "It is what it is," and provides a response to an imperfect world when we feel powerless to achieve Utopia. It is the universal confession that the plea from the Serenity Prayer for God to "grant me the serenity to accept the things I cannot change" has *not* been answered, and we are not willing to accept defeat even after we have given up trying.

In the 1980s, General Motors aired a series of TV ads with the slogan, "Nobody sweats the details like GM." That campaign made a huge impact on me through the years, but I often wondered how true it was. The only thing I could think of then was that people were stressed about matters of quality control that they really cannot do anything about. "Sweating a detail" has all the earmarks of negative emotion without any of the benefits of skillful engineering. It is analogous to someone saying—as many people have, "They can't do anything about your cancer, but I'll pity you."

I wish I had complained with Mr. Henry just a little more. I don't have any answers, but maybe in this case, my complaining in harmony with his suffering would have been a stronger and more helpful sign of compassion and understanding. "Cancer sucks, and these doctors aren't much better!" Maybe it was not true, but maybe it was the sympathizing complaint he needed to hear. After all, whether complaining does any good at all—and I am beginning to think that it does—or whether we can justify complaining against things we cannot do anything about, shouldn't cancer sufferers get a free pass? And shouldn't those who carry the burden of suffering with those patients also get a free pass, with no need to feel guilty about their railing against that bit of reality?

*****

I vowed early after my treatments started that I would not pull the cancer excuse out any more than necessary, whatever "necessary" means. The first time was thrust upon me. I had just turned down a road near our home after we resettled in Michigan. I had maxed out at 41 miles per hour when a police officer pulled me over. He said I was going 6 MPH over the speed limit. I apologized and gave him my license and registration. He looked at it and noticed it was a Wisconsin driver's license.

"Yes, we just moved here," I said.

"What brings you to Michigan?" he interrogated?

""Well," I started, "I was just diagnosed with terminal cancer, and I've come here to die."

The officer strode to his car to make sure that, at least from their legal standpoint, I was legitimate. In a couple minutes, he returned with a look of compassion on his face which, given his young age and profession, he had probably not used yet on the job, and he said, "I'm sorry. Have a good day."

Now I really didn't want to pull that excuse out, because it had very little to do with my reckless, breakneck speeding. But as you can see, his question and my need to answer honestly, forced me into it.

This kind of excuse had become a humorous trope in our family a few years earlier after Caleb was born. Jenn had delightfully used the line, "I just had a baby" up to six or seven years later to justify anything from a missed two-foot putt in golf to being unable to find her car keys. Perhaps it was under her loving inspiration that gave mental airtime to the concept of using my medical condition to merit special treatment. But other than chastising myself for being slow and inept on the tennis court, the only other time I invoked special privilege due to my cancer and its treatment came within months of the speeding incident.

One of the sports I have always enjoyed is ping pong. It was also an activity I considered within my physical reach even while under the throes of chemo. So, shortly after moving back to Michigan, I ordered a table from an Internet table tennis shop and anxiously awaited its arrival. Given that the doctor had given me a statistical terminal date about 5 months past the date I ordered the table, I didn't feel at peace while waiting for it to arrive. At the time, though, there were still supply chain efficiency issues in the aftermath of COVID-19 pressures.

So, I waited. And waited. And after 6 weeks, I received a message that my beautiful table would arrive later in the week. I would have to sign for it since it was big and kind of pricey. Eventually, on Friday I saw this huge delivery truck pull up next to our house. It was still cold with snow on the ground, but I was able to muster the strength and courage to meet the man outside despite my chemo-induced aversion to cold. He pulled out a clipboard and asked me to sign, but only after confirming the condition of the table. In the meantime, he opened the truck, grabbed his industrial pallet jack, and started unloading the table for my examination. But when it came into view, I saw that the box had been punctured, apparently by a forklift. I was concerned. So, we pulled back some cardboard and noticed that a huge gouge was left in the tabletop that rendered it unacceptable. I refused the shipment and contacted the company to start the process over again.

Six weeks later, I was contacted once again that my table would arrive later in the week. Again, on Friday (why is it always late in the week?), a white delivery truck pulled up next to the house. Once again, I held the clipboard while I awaited the opportunity for inspection. And once again, I saw a huge hole puncture in the main surface of the box. Once again, I noticed a long, deep gouge in the table. Oddly, it was not in the same spot as the last one, so I knew they were not just re-sending the same delivery.

This time, when I contacted the company, I suggested they might want to consider another delivery method and pleaded with them that they expedite this next delivery. After all, I mentioned as I tossed out my trump card, I am dying from cancer and I would like to use this table while I can, thank you very much. Two weeks later, a pristine table arrived and we were able to put it in the basement ready to use. As a cherry on top, and maybe since the company was deeply compassionate about my mortal plight, the company granted me a $25 coupon off anything in their store. Unfortunately, there is nothing in their store under $50. Maybe I should've said, "I just had a baby."

*****

As Shaw's serpent illustrates, even if Eden were our world, there might still be conflicting versions of perfection. Even in paradise, life together means that there will always be two or more sets of eyes to see things, two or more hearts to long for things, and two or more stomachs to crave things. Recognizing these differences of priorities and concerns, I am trying to climb the steep learning curve of complaining about things that are not merely a matter of my unique perspective. I try not to complain about other drivers on the road, those that go slower than I do, and those that go faster than I do, knowing that doing so only suggests that I am the gold standard of driving perfection, which I am not. I try not to complain about road construction when the main roads are being worked on for years, and all the alternative routes are also shut down. They are the professionals, and they know what they are doing sometimes. I try not to complain about senseless traffic lights even when I see 50 cars stacked up at red lights and nobody going through the crossroads, because they have surely applied sophisticated artificial intelligence to discover that keeping as many cars on the road as long as possible is the best way to move traffic.

But these lessons about complaining are hard for me. Though I have always hated wasting time at stop lights, being given lots of extra days to live has encouraged me to re-evaluate what time is and what it means to waste time. I am still working hard to understand the blessing that my current life is without complaining that I am not as comfortable or nimble as I used to be. At one point, when I was almost at my weakest, I was outside watching my neighbor, Rick, now a strength and conditioning coach for the University of Alabama, doing some yard work. He was loading a wheelbarrow with debris when a junior sized football came bouncing my way. I grabbed it and, from about 40 feet, I told him I could toss the ball into the wheelbarrow. I mean, I was never a great quarterback, but I used to be able to chuck a football 40 yards easily. Here I was, one third of that distance, feeling pressure to perform before my incredibly strong neighbor and friend. I tossed it and it fell short about ten feet. "Let me try it again!" Attempt number two was better, but still feeble. I was slightly embarrassed, but I knew Rick understood. What surprised me, though, was that I did not complain about it. At least at that moment, I was happy to be alive, and happy to have thrown a ball at all.

We all complain, and most of the time, we shrug off the complaints of others. I recently found myself whining to my tennis colleagues about being unable to perform at the level I want, and I cannot do it without pain. This is a compassionate group, but my gripe was met with an endless stream of all their bodily breakdowns. I realized then as I had realized in the past, that nobody really hears the complaints of others because we all have too many of our own. Even dating back to my junior year in high school, I had knee surgery that ended my basketball playing career, and I remember thinking how much that would change my life. And I somehow created this fantasy that other people would be equally affected by that. But for everybody else, it was just a thing. Somebody else's thing.

So, does that mean that complaining is a useless negative emotional reaction with not a whit of good for anyone? On the contrary. Reflecting on Shaw's and then John Kennedy's inspiring dreaming, while they both can be regarded in broad terms as dissatisfaction about the way things are, to ask the question "Why not?" about a dream for a better future can inspire action and a plan to get us to that better future. We don't need to be resigned to a world in which "It is what it is", but we can express our dissatisfaction in ways that will not settle for cancer's hegemony on us. Or as Jürgen Moltmann writes, "Those who hope in Christ can no longer put up with reality as it is."

The strongest case for a cancer patient's claim to virtuous complaining is that complaining creates an antagonist so we can fight longer. But if we all complain together, as I should have complained with Mr. Henry, we become united in the fight together. None of us can fight this disease alone, but when we complain and put money behind our complaints to cancer-fighting causes, our complaints become a holy force.

9 REJOICING

Rejoice in the Lord always. I will say it again: Rejoice!
– Philippians 4:4

By the third week of April after my initial diagnosis, Dr. Ahmad ordered my chemo treatments to stop. The medically administered beatdown was too severe. Any sense of enjoyment associated with either end of the digestive process had been left in the distant past, and I was becoming dangerously weak. At one point, I was on the couch downstairs and Jenn was holding my hand. "I don't think I can do this anymore. I'm tired, and I hate not being able to function."

She understood better than anyone. She knew the high level of zest that constituted the real me, and she realized that the true version of me no longer existed. It was time for her to act. Since she could do nothing to restore my energy level, she had determined it was time to prepare for the end of my life.

One of Jenn's friends, Mike, a hospice nurse, agreed to visit with me. Our conversation was strange, I remember, because I could not get the questions about the dying procedure out of my mind. He had seen many people whither to nothing, then die. And despite my questions, I really did not want to take part in death. At least not yet. And I was curious about how horrible pancreatic cancer death was, still thinking about my friend's assessment that it was the worst cancer she dealt with among her patients. "Is the pain really awful?" I asked.

Mike's response surprised me. "I once had a patient who had your kind of cancer, and the pain she felt was nothing that a little Tylenol couldn't handle."

Since Tylenol cannot handle mild headaches for me, I was encouraged. But I pressed, "Really? I thought it was much worse!" And in fact, later recollections of my chat with Mike reminded me that he said it usually is much worse, but for the moment, his words soothed my fears.

I pictured myself dying, wondering what it is like on the other side. I embraced the firm but unwilling conviction that eternity is a joyful existence, free from pain, free from sorrow, free from writer's block, free from missed three-foot putts.

I have seen too many people near death. Long before they die, they have already died. I do not want to complain, but I'm sure I will. I want to go out—and I will go out—with rejoicing in my heart as much as I can. I want to beam the confidence that Dietrich Bonhoeffer did at the brutal end of his life: This is the end—for me, the beginning of life.

Mike then related a couple of experiences he had with similar patients. As he spun the narratives, I remember putting myself in his patients' bodies, going through what they were living out, but also begging God not to let any of this experience befall me. Still, I played over in my mind the final scene of my life in which I am drugged beyond consciousness so that I might tolerate the misery: I am no longer aware of those around me; nor am I of myself.

With death scenarios on repeat running through my mind and our conversations, we set up an appointment with the palliative care team from the hospital. As part of their package, their spiritual director agreed to pay a visit. I remember discussing with Jenn where this conversation should take place. I had been confined to the couch for a while because our bedroom was upstairs. Her concern about getting my carcass upstairs was justified. But maybe going upstairs is easier than going downstairs. I'm sure, I thought at the time, I have enough within me to climb thirteen stairs. With that gritty commitment behind me, we arranged to meet the spiritual director of the palliative care team upstairs.

The migration up to the bedroom was not as problematic as I thought it would be. And once a full-time resident in my bedroom, I was close to the bathroom and close to the stockpile of high calorie Pepto-like nutritional drinks Jenn placed next to the bed.

What fascinated me with myself during the director's visit was how I could not suppress my true colors. She came over to talk about end-of-life matters, what I was thinking, whether there was joy in my life, how healthy my faith was, and all that. But all I could think about was that I have someone in my room who has a theological education. Rather than her typical crucial conversation topics, I wanted to ask about her school experience, what part of theological studies she was most passionate about, and did she take this class and that class, courses of study that were possibly ones that I had taught in the past.

I am sure my conversational interests represent at least a significant minority among the dying. Debbie, a good friend of mine from Shawano, told me about a similar conversation her brother had after discovering his cancer was terminal. The chaplain addressed all the important but typical topics to make sure Debbie's brother was able to pass away with peace in his heart. But with blunt honesty, he stated that he would rather have talked about sports.

My daughter, Rachel, was in the area on Friday evening and decided to swing by the house to pay me a visit. It had been weeks since we had seen each other in person, and Jenn showed her up to the room which was my prison. Rachel did an excellent job of hiding her shock at my appearance, which was gaunt and frail, and she spent time reminding me of all the reasons she would not allow me to leave the planet just yet. She promised to return on Sunday to see me again, and that visit was sweet and painful in equal measure since we all shared the unspoken sense that this could be the last time we would enjoy together.

During these visits, Jenn was arranging a photo session to take place with our entire family in the very park where she and I had exchanged our wedding vows. I thought it was a great idea, but I completely hated the thought of appearing in those pictures as if I prepared for an Edvard Munch portrait sitting. Besides, traveling to the park presented a sextuple challenge: Getting back down the stairs, getting into the car at home, getting out of the car, and the reverse of those three actions. The spirit was willing, but the flesh had disappeared from my bones.

Instead of the park, we sculpted plans to take the photos at home in our bedroom. I didn't like this plan, but I was not able to alter its course. I found out later that Jenn called my mother and brothers to join for the photo sitting because she wanted to make sure they could see me one last time. It was evident that my story was writing its conclusion faster than I expected.

Monday dawned another day and my eyes opened. However, I was unable to drink the highly caloric glop that had been my sustenance for days. Water was even too difficult to swallow. Jenn and I lay in bed that night silently. I am sure she was praying for me. And I prayed for her heart to be strong. Jenn had already been a widow once, and this seemed a joke too cruel for God to play on her tender heart again. At some point in the night, I closed my eyes as uncertainty hung in the air whether I would ever open them again.

There is an infinite distance between a difficult task and an impossible one. Tuesday morning my eyes opened. Something was different. Jenn asked what I needed. I replied, "I'm hungry." and I arose from the bed, I walked down the stairs, and I ate.

*****

So, we executed the plan to take pictures in the park. Ideally, we wanted to have the pictures in the pavilion where we were married, but the seventy feet or so to get to the pavilion from our parking space was insurmountable for my emaciated body. I remembered apologizing for needing help to get out of the car, and I remember the kind patience of everyone in my family and the kindness of Jenn's photographer friend, Kathi, who had volunteered to shoot the photos and produce the prints as a lovely parting gift.

I smile in these pictures, but I don't like either my smile or the pictures. I see love in everyone's face, and the faces all have smiles. But these smiles have the pall of "he was a good man when he was alive" on them. The smiles are not fake, but very clearly, they all celebrate what had been rather than what lay ahead. My smile especially, because of my health, is painted on my skull with a layer of flesh akin to a coat of Ultrawhite latex paint. I remember when smiling, I tried to project the joy that defined my life, hoping they would all remember when smiles were easy, springing from the same belly that gave birth to uproarious laughter. That laughter was to be part of my legacy, but this manufactured smile was my attempt to rejoice.

In our emotional lives, we are often unable to rejoice, not because we don't *want* to rejoice, but because there are other emotions in the way. I know this was very much the case for Jenn. I know it was true for me as well. It is hard to rejoice when our hearts are full of anger. It is hard to rejoice when the future is ominously in question. The dread of sadness is strong enough to silence joy. I asked myself how is it possible to experience joy? I wondered if I would be excused if I did not even want to.

Until the words, "I'm hungry," came out of my mouth, I had grown single-mindedly philosophical about the place of happiness or fulfillment or rejoicing in my life when I perceived life as ebbing away. But surely, there is something in all my pastoral training, in all those sessions sitting with other people who have suffered, yet smiled, and from my reading in theology and in Scripture. I knew the wisdom those experiences communicated, and I had mined it and served up gold nuggets to various listeners, passionate or indifferent, who comprised my Sunday morning pew-bound audience. But now it was time for me to contextualize theory and find a way to rejoice when I'm physically and emotionally destitute.

I would like to say that I had found the spiritual depth to rejoice in my suffering. At least I knew how to define joy. Joy is not the simple absence of sadness. Joy is not happiness. Joy is not optimism. Michael J. Fox's memoir talks about his "particularly bad year" of 2018 when his optimism ran out. And he starts thinking about mortality. Optimism is the belief that everything will work out great in the future, but Fox points out that at some point, you run out of Future. That is precisely where I found myself.

So, with my future ostensibly dwindling, I started looking for opportunities to get to the next moment with joy in my heart because the big picture is bleak, and the big miracle is not guaranteed. That turning point, when I said, "I'm hungry," was the first moment in the whole cancer experience Jenn and I found that we could share rejoicing together.

One stratagem that held promise to pump joy into my heart was to look for little victories. Maybe it is less chilly outside than yesterday. My mind is still sharp and aware. My kids are closer to me than ever. And I recalled that moment just a few weeks ago when I knocked in a golf shot from 75 yards out.

Regardless of how I felt on the inside, I tried to project a rejoicing heart on the outside. It must have worked a little bit. Our neighbor, Rick, saw me outside one afternoon, and I recall him saying, "For a man in your condition, you sure seem happy." I think I was faking it, but maybe it was from decades of having lots to be happy about. And why not? The sun was shining, and I am still here!

Part of my rejoicing stems from my love of a challenging fight. I remember when the discussions were taking place within the medical reports as to whether my cancer was everywhere, or whether the lesions on my liver were confirmed as cancer, that I silently screamed, "Bring it on!" I never specifically hoped that it was everywhere, but if it was going to be there, let's bring it. Half of that was hopelessness, knowing that it may not matter much, anyway, with my kind of cancer. But the other half of my emotional response was knowing that the victory, when it comes, will be a greater one.

I often wonder about the parameters of rejoicing. Does rejoicing happen because reality is better than expected? Is it the opposite of complaining which only happens when reality is less than expected? I confess that I can complain even when life is good, so should I have learned that rejoicing is not limited by a contrast between the way things are and the way you want them to be? As Paul invites us to rejoice in the Lord always, I try to imagine how I can make joy a reality that is always present.

I found myself thinking about the earliest Christians and how they must have talked often about rejoicing. I have no idea what it would have been like to experience a community of faith whose past began within the last generation or two. Christians today, like many Americans, assume the future is guaranteed because the past is so massive.

However they thought about the church's future, the struggle for its survival was woven into the fabric of the daily lives of those first Christians. When Paul tells the Roman church to rejoice with those who rejoice, his advice comes with a certain backdrop of suffering and persecution. He tries to strengthen the solidarity of the faith community there knowing that there are others in the region who will bring persecution and strife. It makes good sense, from an emotional point of view, that he encourages them to rejoice whenever they get the chance, whether it is for their own personal celebration, or someone else's.

Thus, it also makes good sense from an emotional point of view for my friends and family, acquaintances and strangers, those of you who wept with my illness, to rejoice together with me in my rejoicing. So many of my friends, and my family, even new people I did not know well, rejoiced with me. This is your victory, too, Rick. And Andrew. And Drew. Dear friends at Shawano, you pulled me through. Shelley, Keith, and Jim, this victory is yours! Please rejoice with me, too. And my hope is that we spread this widening web of mutual celebration.

10 LIVING

DEAD PERSON: I'm not dead!
MORTICIAN: Here -- he says he's not dead!
CUSTOMER: Yes, he is.
DEAD PERSON: I'm not!
MORTICIAN: He isn't.
CUSTOMER: Well, he will be soon, he's very ill.
DEAD PERSON: I'm getting better!
– from "Monty Python and the Holy Grail"

Yet, the tumor was still there. Still wrapped around every major artery and vein. Still choking the hope that I had that something was going to change. Still taunting me to give up. The tumor was still there.

In the short time since diagnosis, Jenn and I had become experts in our own minds at reading the various reports dropped into my patient portal. From the first CT scan in December 2020 until today when the latest scan popped into my portal, we were left with words describing what evil things had shifted, moved, or (hopefully) disappeared. We pieced together the picture of my insides to determine if we should laugh or weep or maybe both.

It was July and I had been feeling a little better. The effects of chemo waned. I was enjoying time with my family and trying to make the most of what little time I had left. My Oncology Radiologist, Dr. DiCarlo, had warned me that the effects of the targeted radiation may shrink the tumor growing in my pancreas some and it may give me a little more time to live, and so it seemed worth a shot. I wanted more time even if I could only get a little.

In the quest for more time, seeing this scan devastated us. Not a millimeter's change in the size of the growth in my pancreas. Jenn and I braced ourselves for the worst as we walked into the Oncology office. The radiation had not worked. There were no more options. There was no more time.

We sat in the chairs in Dr. Ahmad's office silently, waiting for him to enter, draped in his executioner's cloak to deliver the final blow. With no more options, I imagined the words coming out of his mouth as I sat there numbly, "We'll do everything we can to keep you comfortable...." I heard them like I was in a dream. How can you hear those words and how can they have any meaning at all? This is not the outcome I expected. Or maybe it was. I can no longer remember what we expected from any of this. Yet, I was sure the tumor was still there.

After what seemed like an eternity in Hell's waiting room, Dr. Ahmad entered. With the same spry spring in his step, he asked, "How are you doing today, Lew?" A small smile stretched across his lips as he sat down on his stool and typed into his computer and pulled up the chart, ready to read the verdict and deliver the death sentence.

I do not know how I answered him. I may not have answered at all.

"You had a scan after your radiation and let's see what it says" started the doctor. "Oh, what is this?"

I held my breath. My ears remained closed as I wept to myself. "I know. No change. The tumor is still there."

Dr. Ahmad continued. "It looks like the tumor is dead."

"The tumor is dead?" I managed to eke out. I assumed "dead" in this context was some kind of ironic medical terminology that deflected the victim's obsession with painful reality.

"Yes. The scan says, 'necrotic fluid filled mass.' The tumor is dead. The lymph nodes are clear, and the liver is clear as well. I see no evidence of cancer."

I looked at Jenn. We were holding hands expecting the news no one ever wants to receive. Instead, the doctor delivered good news that no one ever expects. I looked at the doctor. "What does this mean?"

"We can't say there is no cancer, but we can't find any right now." said Dr. Ahmad.

"So, what do I do now?"

"Go live your life. I will see you in three months after your next scan. We'll just keep monitoring and see what happens. This is great news!"

We walked out of the office with our arms around each other. Tears streamed down our faces. We got into the car and cried together. "What just happened in there?" I asked.

"We just got your life back," Jenn said.

And so, I lived.

*****

Before the appointment with Dr. Ahmad, we had planned a summer farewell tour of things I loved: Trips to see my beloved White Sox, art museums, The Rocket Mortgage Classic golf tournament, and other places and events that aligned with my passions. We wanted to enjoy these things while I was still alive, but we assumed they would be the last such things we would do together. When my death sentence turned into a life sentence once again, each pre-planned farewell turned into a celebration of what might be possible now.

But the change of perspective did nothing to help me shift back into the process of living. I have stated before that my formula for living had always been to prepare for something and then do that something. But after Dr. Ahmad's good news, I confronted the oddest challenge of my entire life: Life lay in front of me, but I had not *prepared* to live again. I was adrift in a sea of blessedness, and I did not know how to recover. Improvisation was never my strength, so I tried to lay hold of a plan, but there was no plan.

Sure, it was great to enjoy ball games and golf tournaments, but those events are distractions from life, not life itself. I needed to dig back into life if my borrowed time on which I lived was to have any significance.

That is why I always hated the movie, "The Bucket List." I understand the sentiment, but I always thought that living only for enjoyment, at any stage of life, is a little bit cheap. I once knew a woman whose terminal diagnosis inspired her to leap headlong into wall-to-wall partying until she could no longer get outside of the house. She had no heirs, so banks who delivered credit cards financed her bacchanalia. I asked her what happens if she outlives her credit limit. "Don't worry," she replied. "I won't." Again, I get the sentiment, but I needed a plan in sync with my view of life in the world.

The main thing for me was getting back to life as I understood its deepest and best sense, so I could not focus on its distractions. With new days of life to look forward to, I wanted to do meaningful and enjoyable things without the gloom of immediate death souring every experience. But this is simply a desire, not a plan. What if I do not need a plan at all?

*****

Physically, we, the living, are closer to the grave than we were yesterday. And whether we think about it or not, that transition from being alive to being dead is always happening. Religions often try to help us in that transition, making us ready for whatever comes next, and often puts lots of treats and incentives along our paths to make sure that the transition and the outcome are as favorable as possible. In a way, these treats and incentives are the plan we execute to transition to whatever is next.

Indeed, religions often talk about the transition from death to life, but this is usually thought of in symbolic terms. The epigraph of this book from the gospel of John ("they have gone from death to life") seems to be one of those symbolic statements on first blush. But John's story is much messier than that. There is evidence that John's faith community believed Jesus' words in John 11 literally when he said, "I am the resurrection and the life," but that these two groups of people were separate. "People who believe in me will live even if they die, and everyone who lives and believes in me will never die!" This is a great comfort if you can get everyone around you to embrace it, but what happens, as is likely the case in John's church group, if people whose faith is beyond question start to die? John's faith community's response to the reality of physical death is reflected in Jesus' declaration of being both the resurrection and the life.

So, the language of going from death to life in John 5:24, even if it mainly a metaphor for living authentically and faithfully for God, at least recognizes the desire to transition from a life that is physically ebbing away to one that is transitioning the other way. In my own experience, having a physical life that has been returned to me gives me insights into the literal side of that transition that I did not perceive before my diagnosis and successful treatments.

One of the biggest insights for me was that I had become anesthetized to the transition from life to death while simultaneously being unaware of the ongoing transition back to life. The cancer diagnosis surprised me, and the successful treatments surprised me. But I have started to embrace those surprises as the miracles they are. Most people, I fear, get used to living so the miracle of life is lost to them.

Five months after the startling optimistic scan result was interpreted by Dr. Ahmad, when a friend asked us to attend his church's Christmas Eve service, we were singing a Christmas carol with the congregation when I was overwhelmed with unspeakable joy because of the life that had been given to me by the grace of God and by the amazing application of science. The tears of joy I shed that night would reappear every couple of days between then and now. But the question for me becomes why I did not periodically erupt with tears of joy before my cancer diagnosis. It is because I had gotten used to living, spoiled by the normalcy of life. I suppose I need to give myself a little grace in this, but it is unfortunate that we only awaken to the reality that everything is precious, including our sense of life's value, and how quickly it can all go away, when we or someone we love has it put in jeopardy. Until that happens, most of us are unaware of transitioning to anything else because we think we are already dead—physically or spiritually—or alive—physically or spiritually, and we cannot see any alternative to our current state.

Even now, as I embrace the miracle of where I am going from where I was, I can do better. Sure, I have prayed, but others have prayed more faithfully. I have tried to embrace hope, but others were more hopeful. I have tried to express gratitude when life appears, but I am often grumpy because unimportant stuff—things like joint pain from immunotherapy, or numbness in my feet from chemo, or muscle weakening from old age—are a regular part of my daily life. "That's OK," I remind myself. It is OK by way of the blessedness of living against all odds, but it is not OK because I am often oblivious to the miracle that is my life. Yes, I can do better, and I will do better as I try to live up to the hopeful ideals that I proclaim in my life story.

What I cannot do is pretend that I am any kind of hero. I am often embarrassed at how passive I am while receiving unexpected miracles, one after the next. I feel like a modern-day Lazarus. His story was the subject of my doctoral dissertation, so I already feel like he is my brother in the life-death-life journey. He is the guy that died, apparently because Jesus took his sweet time to pay him a healing visit only to bring him back to life when everyone else thought his corpse would be in a smelly state of decomposition.

Lazarus is the perfect non-heroic hero. While people around him are weeping and complaining, he is safely tucked away in his tomb without a worry in the world. Eventually, Jesus prays demonstratively and works a life renewing miracle. He orders Lazarus to come out of the tomb which the formerly dead man does, accomplishing the only action attributed to him in the story. Yes, that is me! I have done nothing to benefit from this miracle, but I am a passive recipient of this grace. The only thing I do, I do faithfully: I exit the tomb.

*****

If people are faithful to their instincts, in the story world of Lazarus, I can see skeptics gather around him to pounce on how incomplete his remarkable recovery was. And if Lazarus' portrayal is faithful to human biology, he eventually dies. Then the skeptics march in, claiming that his miracle is no miracle at all. The skeptics who discount miracles want to discount this one because the man who was dead and then alive, is dead once again.

Does this mean that my story is not miraculous because I still must deal with treatments and concerns for recurrence? Does that mean that my story is less hopeful, even if I am gone before you have read this story?

Until then, I wonder if I will ever become indifferent to this continuous stream of miracles. Put another way, is it possible to embrace the transition from life to whatever is next while still embracing the miracle of my current life? As it stands now, from life to life sounds wonderful. I always want more.

That is not a position shared by everyone. A few days before he died, Jenn's grandpa said, "I've lived a good long life. I'm tired and I miss my Little Darlin'." He was almost 92. I wondered if I would ever be in a situation where those would be my words or if the greed for more life would persist. The story of Hezekiah, when he was granted a stay of expiration, giving him fifteen more years to live simply reminded me that fifteen more years for me would still be decades away from the one hundred and ten years I promised to Caleb and Jenn. Then, at age 110, would that be enough? Mustn't life end?

Aristotle said a story has three parts: a beginning, a middle, and an end. But he was only two-thirds right. Sometimes, a story, as we tell it, has no end. We are all living in the middle.

11 DYING AGAIN AND LIVING AGAIN

I runne to death, and death meets me as fast,
And all my pleasures are like yesterday.
– John Donne, *Holy Sonnet I*

There are two ways: One of life, and one of death. And there
is a huge difference between the two ways.
– The Didache

"If everything looks good in August, we can talk about taking your
chemo port out." Thus spake Dr. Ahmad.

After two years of walking on broken glass, we were so close to a
finish line. I love a good competition, but now it felt like the
unlikely victory we hoped for was in our grasp. This was a
monumental dream taking shape before us. We bounced out of Dr.
Ahmad's office dancing on clouds. Just three more months and the
last vestige of this awful disease would be removed from my chest,
and I would be free of the memories of the past three years.

My blood test two days before that August appointment would
take us down a different path, though. The downward trend of my
CA 19-9 reversed course and trended upward once again. The CT
scan showed some "concerning" lymph nodes in my celiac chain

on both my left and right sides and a few "enlarged" lymph nodes were cautionary around my pancreas. An appointment that should have ended in scheduling the removal of a chemo port concluded with scheduling a PET scan instead.

In the interim, we resolved to keep living. Rachel called me and asked if I wanted to go to London for a weekend in September. The tickets were affordable, and it was a once-in-a-lifetime opportunity. Jenn already had a business trip to Florida planned that weekend, and under the weight of Jenn's and Rachel's insistence, I knew I would have to expend Herculean strength to refuse this invitation. Should I seize the moment (carpe diem and all that), or retreat to my safe and boring normal existence?

While considering this invitation, I thought about Miss Edna. Many years earlier, while youth director at my first church job, I performed visitation duties while the lead pastor was on vacation. During my weekly rounds, I saw Edna, a lovely homebound woman who clearly needed more company than she received. I was surprised and delighted at the beauty and energy of our time together. In those days, I didn't know how to terminate a conversation, so I stayed for well over an hour. She invited me back, and I willingly promised to make a return visit. What I was less willing or able to do was fulfill the promise while I had the opportunity. I was busy with family, with school, with softball leagues, and any number of valid and invalid excuses. Plus, I committed myself to directing a highly successful youth group. Besides, I would be able to see her when there was a break in my schedule. However, that break never came. I learned that she died in the early fall. I learned that opportunities need to be embraced with action, not promises. So, with Rachel's invitation on the table, not only did I *promise* to travel with her, but I also bought actual tickets and turned steadfastly toward London and all its Nigels and Geoffreys-with-a-G and colours-with-a-u and beans for breakfast.

The PET scan was cautionary. The results would arrive while we were on our trips, and we were pretty sure the results were good. All indications suggested that cancer was part of my history, not my future. I remember sharing afternoon tea with Rachel in London and telling her my excitement but also shared with her that Jenn and I agreed to wait until we returned from our trips to look at the results. We had experienced all the big moments of this journey together, and we did not want this one to be any different. Besides, we were confident the lymph nodes were simply a little angry for one reason or another and ready to settle down any minute now. The weekend in London was well worth the fatigue of traveling halfway around the world twice in 4 days. Jenn returned sun-kissed from Florida and I road-weary from London, and it was time to read the results. My heart raced as we clicked to login to my patient portal. There seemed to be an eternity of clicks to get to the test results we were looking for, but once we navigated to the page, I didn't want to click on the bold highlighted unseen report. I hesitated. Jenn put her hand on my shoulder and squeezed gently to give me the strength to click.

There it was, in black and white, in ones and zeros, in simple English words. Cancer: Yes. I looked at Jenn and back at the screen. I asked, "What does it mean?" Not because I didn't understand the results, but because I couldn't believe the results. Jenn held me and said, "I'm sorry." There was nothing else to say. What we thought was going to be a time to celebrate was marred once again by the threat of pancreatic cancer coming back to try to finish the job it failed so miserably at the first time.

Pancreatic Cancer recurs in patients about 89% of the time. Surviving for 2 years from a stage 4 diagnosis without any surgery is a statistic almost too small to calculate. Surviving stage 4 cancer 2 times is statistically not even registered. There just are not enough cases to have statistics.

We entered the doctor's office once again prepared for the worst, but honestly, we were hopeful that I could defy the odds again. I had made it through the initial round. I survived my stomach perforation. How bad could pancreatic cancer 2.0 be, really?

Dr. Ahmad's normally spry step and small smile were somewhat muted as he entered the room. "How are you doing, Lew?" Just like always.

"You tell me, Doctor," I said.

He went on to tell me I had cancer again, which I knew. He began to rattle off treatment options and courses of action and so many words that just turned into a Charlie Brown cartoon of muted noises of adults to children.

There was a break in the cacophony, and I asked, "So, Dr. Ahmad, what does this mean? What are my chances?" I heard every word with crystal clarity.

"If treatment goes well, maybe four to six months."

I don't remember anything else from that visit.

Jenn and I stumbled down the hall and out to the car. This time, we efficiently managed the effusion of tears, either through our experience in cancer-induced emotions, or through pain-induced emotional anesthetization. "Did he say four to six months?" I asked.

"I don't see how that is possible!" Jenn replied. "Look at you. You are healthy and active and there is nothing wrong with you! You play tennis 3 times a week and golf every day. How can they say you're going to be gone in 4-6 months?"

We drove home in silence.

Breaking the news to the kids was painful. Rachel, Josh, and Caleb all seemed to be in disbelief. We had all taken good news as the only news, so this news was particularly difficult to hear. After the initial shock of the turn of events wore off, Jenn went into planning mode.

She decided that waiting for me to decline was a bad plan for pictures and scheduled them for the week before I started chemo. Josh flew up from Dallas to visit that week; Rachel, Alex, and the kids drove over, and we took beautiful photos at the peak of fall in our neighborhood. It was a much better photo experience than the last time we all gathered for photos, but I've learned to associate pictures with the last thing I might ever do. Dear God, I hate pictures!

We also prepared a mid-October Thanksgiving celebration just in case I was unable to taste food by the real Thanksgiving. Jenn can tell you the complications and difficulties of trying to find turkey at a reasonable price outside of the month of November, but we had a beautiful meal full of delicious food and the best company I could dream of in the whole world. The only problem with the meal was that after it, I had to start chemo. Again.

We pulled into the Infusion Center for my first treatment. It had been so long since I had been in this place for this reason. Thankfully, COVID precautions were mainly a thing of the past and that meant that Jenn could accompany me to my infusion appointments. These infusions would also be much shorter and easier on my body. At least that was the theory. But at the end of the day, the less effective chemo was just that: Less effective. Not only was the treatment *less* effective; it was not effective in any way at all. After one round, the score was pancreatic cancer: 100; Lew: 0. I was bald again. I was tired all the time. My life was shrinking, and the cancer was growing. I realized that if I had started with this chemo treatment in the beginning, I would not be writing this book at all.

Our meeting with Dr. Ahmad after round one led to the switch in treatment to immunotherapy as the only treatment. A newer treatment for pancreatic cancer patients, Keytruda, an immunotherapy particularly helpful in those with Lynch Syndrome, would be administered every three weeks. We would see if this would affect the march of cancer through my abdomen. After the first three treatments, we were ready to start evaluating the effectiveness of the protocol. The first positive indicator was the blood test. My CA 19-9 came in as Jenn and I were driving to an appointment with Dr. Raus. I clicked open the test results while we were on the road. It was time to rip the Band-Aid off. After almost 3 years, the number was in the green section of the graph. It was in the *normal* range! Being normal never felt so good.

I'm pretty sure Jenn almost wrecked the car, but somehow, she got us safely pulled off to the side of the road so she could see for herself. There it was. *Normal.* Immunotherapy was working.

*****

Even in survival, cancer changes us. Cancer and all our current treatments will never leave us better than we have ever been, physically. The theoretically maximal result is that we are not worse than when we started. More likely is the outcome that treatments damage us in ways that will never leave.

As one who always met the challenge of aging head on, I have always smugly enjoyed being able to compete with athletes less than half my age. Sure, there were losses in quickness, strength, and agility, but increases in experience, wisdom, and cageyness kept me in the game.

Cancer's physical toll on my abilities to function normally are hard to define. In part, one of the things that make it so hard to know what cancer has done to me is that the aftermath of treatments run parallel to the normal decline from aging. These losses now far outpace whatever improvements I can ever add through cleverness acquired from age. But still, I hope.

When I watch Josh play volleyball, I wonder if we could still form a topflight father-son duo. We played together in a tournament several years ago and I still love wearing the championship T-shirt. But the calendar year printed on the shirt suggests that the tournament success is not as recent as it seems that it was.

I recently watched videos of a tournament he played in Florida. During one match, my son's team was playing poorly. I found myself hypothetically suggesting that I could have come in as Josh's partner and we could have been successful again. But then I reminded myself that just a couple months earlier, we played some pickup volleyball together locally against a couple men, a father son combination, over whom I would have expected to prevail. That is, I would have expected us to prevail under normal circumstances. But normal circumstances are a part of the past for me. [Jenn, the editor, informs the reader that this other father-son team was an average of 18 years younger than the Lew-Josh team. Lew, the author, reminds the reader and the editor that this information is irrelevant.] Even the concept of a "new normal", the idea that life's changing landscape makes a return to yesterday impossible, for better or for worse, and I must learn to adjust, was not enough to dispel my temptation to compare normals. In my current situation, immunotherapy had rendered my joints and muscles, and nearly any movement that uses them—which includes all movements—problematic. Had I really stepped into the court with Josh at the Florida tournament, we would not win.

In my post-cancer life, I see my positive contributions in volleyball fading, even more quickly than what would happen through age alone. I will still go and watch Josh play, usually some local leagues and tournaments, and I always hope his team will need a sub and I can step in. But there is a time I must stop imagining that I am still twenty-something and cancer free. Jenn looks at me and asks, "When will you stop doing that?"

I will stop doing that, but not for a while. Indeed, there will be a future when Josh plays volleyball, Rachel travels overseas on a whim, Jenn sees a movie with Caleb, and all these things will happen, and I cannot join them. It happens to everyone, and contrary to popular grumbling, the reason is even more unavoidable than taxes. But that future is not now.

For all of us, the future is uncertain, in terms both of length and direction. Many of us who are victims of cancer would like to determine the direction of our life even if we know its length is affected. What I work on every day now is to make my life's direction as beautiful as possible. I confess, though, that this is an ideal that is hard to accomplish when cancer is always working to affect its length.

What I want, what nearly every cancer victim wants, is permanence. We want treatments to work like antibiotics, kicking cancer and all its possibilities of returning away forever. I love that Dr. Ahmad has recently told us that I am in "complete remission," a phrase I had lusted over and expressed jealousy toward even while still celebrating its owners' blessed health.

I was recently looking at my new CA 19-9 numbers, and the result caused me some trouble. The numbers were still in the normal range because of immunotherapy's success. But there has been a slight trend in the wrong direction. I am not a doctor, and I do not know how to make an intelligent evaluation, but I do know, through years of practice, how to worry about stuff like this. And that is apparently what I chose to do that night.

Doctors will ask me how I'm doing. I know what they're really asking: They want to know how I am feeling so their medical palliative instincts can be applied. But what I want to say is that my answer depends wholly on how my chances of survival are going. The hardest adjustment I ever had to make was learning to live for the moment. I had to start living as if there were no tomorrow after decades of believing that there would be tens of thousands more tomorrows.

*****

When I look at the future and all its tomorrows, I realize that life is like watching a toy boat drift away from a pond's shore. While we live, we hold the boat in our hands and do whatever we can to prepare it for its Forever journey. Then, at some point, the craft drifts away, carried by the unpredictable nudging of the waters. Our influence is gone, but we are still concerned spectators.

But on the Forever voyage, there is a bigger pond, and the winds will not return the boat to us. It continues to drift, and eventually, long past our reach, the boat is unseen by us. Others we have known, people who have loved us and saw us build our boat, people who were inspired by our boat and who helped and inspired us, will watch it drift. And if we have built a good vessel, they will retrieve the boat, and remember our craftsmanship, and appreciate it, and continue to sail it in the pond.

One day, our days are done, and others will only be able to use the pieces of our boat to make one of their own.

EPILOGUE

Had I been present at the Creation, I would have given some useful hints for the better ordering of the universe.
– Attributed to Alfonso X, "The Wise" King of Spain (1221–1284)

I was golfing a round by myself, quickly strolling through the first three holes. But I noticed a lone player along the sixth fairway looking for a ball in the rough. It did not seem likely that he would delay my progress, even if he continued to look for several more minutes. Since nobody else was on the course between us, I stole occasional glances ahead to see how he marched on. Eventually, he either found his ball or gave up looking for it and drove his cart directly to the eighth tee, maybe to speed things along.

After hitting a couple decent drives and finishing the next four holes well enough to give the illusion that I knew what I was doing, I came to the eighth tee. As I drove up, the wizened man who had looked for the ball minutes earlier scooted to the side and flicked his index finger in such a way that I could not tell if a fly was buzzing his head or if he wanted me to play through. I made my way beside him and noticed a distinct and strong cigarette smell emanating from his clothes.

"You can play through," he offered. "I'm pretty slow. I have lung cancer. I've had it for two years."

With this succinct introduction, he managed to introduce himself, push me forward, inspire compassion within me, invite me to share two sentences of my biography, and form an ad hoc brotherhood between us.

"Pancreatic," I responded. "Three and a half years."

I silently prayed for this man and offered what may have sounded like insincere tripe: "Be blessed," I exclaimed ere I drove out of sight, really hoping, in some way, that he would be.

What lingered after this moment of fellowship, other than the cigarette smoke that migrated to my own clothes, was the idea that *pancreatic cancer* and *three and a half years* of survival are not often paired together. The unlikelihood of my survival and relative health have often amazed and puzzled me. And when friends and family suggested I write about my cancer experience and survival so far, my initial question was whether my story resonates with anyone else's story. They adjured me, "Just tell your inspiring story," without really explaining how that inspiration stuff all works. So, in telling my story, I tried hard not to preach, even though I have been a preacher. I have tried hard not to lecture, even though I have been a lecturer. So, I am just telling my story, describing my experience occasionally in painful detail, reflecting my determination, my support, and my growth as a person through it all. How that might help anyone else I will leave to you, Dear Reader, to figure out.

One other issue I have wrestled with while writing this account is how it might end or how it should end. Autobiographies are always incomplete because writing them requires, at the very least, that the author be alive. Therefore, there is always more that *could be* told. Especially when the author battles cancer, it seems that the book's end and the author's end might lie very closely together. After my diagnosis that cancer was found in the lymph nodes, I could not write for months. I did not know how to end the book because I did not know how the story of my life would end.

In a biological sense, none of us achieve victory over death permanently. We cancer survivors know this, but maybe we can celebrate enough victories against our cellular intruder that our cause of death will not be directly related to cancer. We win lots of tiny battles along the way and confront factors that we and our support teams cannot often predict or control. But even when we subdue our foe for a season, like God's word to Cain about sin, cancer "is lurking at the door; its desire is for you." Recurrence is a story we have all heard too many times in the lives of people whose victory seemed to be at hand. Churchill's words seem apt here: Defeat is never fatal. Victory is never final. It's courage that counts.

So, I ask myself in what sense can I ever claim victory over the antagonist of my story? It is always a lifelong battle where victory after victory does not keep cancer from lurking at the door. My responsibility as a patient is to fight as well as I can while embracing the beauty of life. But in the grand picture, to paraphrase Doctor Cox in the sitcom, "Scrubs", everything my care team does to restore health is a stall.

I do not know how close cancer is to my door. Sometimes, the possibility of recurrence feels palpable. I can hear it lurking, panting, slobbering. Sometimes, I give it no thought at all because I feel the beast skulking away with its pointed tail between its legs. But even when optimism is high, my suspicions are strong enough that I hate looking at the results of scans or blood tests. I don't mind NOT hearing the medical news because of that fearful suspicion. I'm like a child at bedtime who, when hearing a scary noise, finds protection under the unassailable armor of a blanket.

I find joy in the battle and I find a sense of victory in being able to fight. I was always moved by Dylan Thomas's poem, "Do Not Go Gentle into that Good Night". Thomas encourages his dying father to "Rage, rage against the dying of the light," a sentiment I have embraced with tears, clenched teeth, and grit in my fight for survival. But whenever I think of these words, I also remember the question asked by my friend, the same one who judged pancreatic cancer as the worst in her professional experience. She asked, "Why not go gentle into that good night?" She hated seeing people suffer as they fade away and she saw a certain dignity in "going gentle". But I see the poem from the heart of a man who knows he is going to miss his father. It is not that he wants to see him suffer, but please, just hang on longer so we can have more time!

It is for more time that I continue my fight. More time to play. More time to complain. More time to rejoice. More time with my family. More time just to see what is next.

*****

Since my initial diagnosis in 2020, one question has dominated my thinking when I try to make sense of it all: What's next? When treatments started, I desperately needed to know how my body would respond. I wanted to know how long treatments would be effective if they were effective at all. I wanted to know the collateral damage these treatments brought. I wanted to know how much additional time the treatments would give me. I wanted to know what other options were available.

Then, after the treatments showed a remarkable level of success and my life could return to a remarkably high level of normalcy, I was left with the same question: What's next? I have unexpected life and health back, but what do I do now? My response cannot be as simple as "keep doing what you're doing" or "stay the course" or anything that assumes past habits and routines will apply to the days ahead. There are certainly common features between the past, the present, and the future. But the rules of the game of life have changed, along with its goals and range of outcomes.

I am responsible for providing some answers to this question. What will I do now? I will play tennis, I will love my family, I will encourage a friend, I will help a stranger, I will write a book. But answers are often out of my control. Tomorrow is never certain, and few people sense this fact more than cancer patients. Whether we embrace the depth of grace of each new day, we know that the days we have ahead of us are not endless. But embracing the grace of new life, new health, and unlikely hope helps me realize that victories are no less miraculous even if those victories are not permanent.

*****

Last week I seized an opportunity to travel back to Shawano. I looked forward to visiting some friends and colleagues, but because of the impromptu nature of the trip, I could not develop a plan to visit all my friends or to directly thank all those who mean so much to me as I journey forward, living this life of unlikely hope. I visited with Shelley at the church, who celebrated the fact that I was standing before her as proof of God's reality.

I also made a special effort to see Joel, whose text to me almost two years ago provided my incentive to begin authoring this story. We celebrated the recent success of the volleyball team I had coached for only one year, but whose strong leadership under Danny, my assistant head coach at the time, guided them to the state finals.

Joel then told me that the high school christened the tournament we host each September the "Abby Tuma Invitational." Her spirit, love of volleyball, and inspiration have made an eternal impact on my life, and I am grateful that her legacy will live on through this recognition.

As for me, I often wonder what my legacy will be. I told some friends just today that I have always tried to live so that a thousand people come to my funeral. But it would be hard for me to verify that I have met my goal. Instead, I consider another, more meaningful legacy: To offer hope for life, as unlikely as it is, in the face of anything.

ACKNOWLEDGMENTS

I am aware, while writing these words of gratitude, that there is more to this book than words. From start to finish, others have inspired me, guided me, encouraged me, loved me, and kept me alive. Many of these people appear in the story, but many more do not. To list them all by name would be a social blunder second only to claim to have gotten the list complete. Forgive me, therefore, if I simply summarize 99% of my gratitude to acknowledging those who have inspired me, guided me, encouraged me, loved me, kept me alive, and played tennis with me.

The other 1% are most important: I am grateful to my family, and especially to Jenn who tells me daily that the world needs me. And I am grateful to Abby who stood with me when she herself could not stand.

ABOUT THE AUTHOR

Lew Worthington is a passionate pastor, father, husband, and friend. He recently converted his commitment to physical and academic excellence to skills at navigating the unknown through his ongoing conflict with cancer. With a PhD from Vanderbilt University in New Testament Studies, Lew has served as a seminary professor, pastor, elder, and teacher in the church. He can be found most days, regardless of the weather, on the tennis court or the golf course. He is most committed these days to spreading his unlikely hope to the ones in front of him. He and his wife, Jennifer, have a talented teenager together, and Lew has 2 grown children as well as 2 grandchildren.

www.ingramcontent.com/pod-product-compliance
Lightning Source LLC
Chambersburg PA
CBHW020939090426
42736CB00010B/1190